PSYCHOANALYTIC INQU

A Topical Journal for Mental Health Professionals

| Volume 26 | 2006 | Number 2 |

Love (and Hate) With the Proper Stranger: Affective Honesty and Enactment:
A Study of Relational Sensibility
Case Presentation and Commentaries

Prologue

This issue of *Psychoanalytic Inquiry* follows a design that has achieved increasing popularity in today's pluralist world of psychoanalytic theory and practice. Providing a case presentation that incorporates detailed process notes along with a number of discussions of that case taken from divergent theoretical perspectives that appeals to the clinician operating in a postmodern setting. By proposing alternative ideas to the reader, the reader is afforded an opportunity to conceptualize from his or her own perspective the approach most conducive to good analytic work for the particular patient as he or she has envisioned her from reading the material presented. Or the reader may discover that alternative views suggested in the discussions may be integrated, establishing a more textured, more complex vision of the analytic pair at work together, a process facilitated through application of a systems sensibility. The abiding lesson—that there is no one good way to do our work but, on the other hand, that not all ways are equally good—is put forward persuasively in this format.

In this issue, Holly Levenkron offers us a clear example of an application of a relational framework to psychoanalysis, presenting an intimate, highly personal view of dramatic engagement with her patient, Ali. She encompasses in her work, as well as in her own commentary on it, illustrations of the concepts of those relationalists who have most influenced her, including Jessica Benjamin, Darlene Ehrenberg, and many of the discussants who share this issue with Dr. Levenkron, including Phillip Bromberg, Stuart Pizer, Malcolm Slavin, and Owen Renik. We are also introduced to Dr. Levenkron's own conceptual contributions to relational psychoanalysis, including her helpful notion of affective honesty, which each of the discussants comments on.

I believe this issue offers another facet of great value to our understanding of what is meant by a relational sensibility. All of the discussants in this issue are relationalists of one form or another, and the very distinctions in their perspectives on Dr. Levenkron's clinical understanding attests to the individuality of all relational thinking. There is no unified relational theory, but there is to be seen in the variety of relational approaches presented here a certain common sensibility—a sensibility that values constructivism, interaction, mutuality, intersubjectivity, enactment, nonlinearity, and affectivity, though the meaning of these concepts does vary somewhat depending on the contributor under consideration.

We are very fortunate in our discussants in this Issue, not only for the seriousness with which they engage Dr. Levenkron's case and her own discussion of it but also for the range in their own thinking. The discussants include Phillip Bromberg, James Fosshage, Barbara and Stuart Pizer, Owen Renik, Malcom Slavin, Donnel Stern, and Judy Teicholz. I can assure you that once you read and think about all of the issues raised in this volume, your understanding of what is meant by relational, what is significant in this sensibility, and how it differs from other approaches will be considerably clearer.

Estelle Shane, Ph.D.
Issue Editor

Love (and Hate) With the Proper Stranger: Affective Honesty and Enactment

HOLLY LEVENKRON, L.I.C.S.W.

In this article I illustrate through detailed clinical examples how an impasse may serve as a function of the failure to negotiate recognition. Amid efforts to remain good objects, we often ignore signals that dictate a more forthright and meaningful communication. Subsequently, patient and analyst are often waylaid in power struggles or in dissociated and deadened moments that detour the achievement of deeper meaning between them. To maintain authenticity in the dyad, the analyst can attempt to speak in honest and forthright ways that embody the analyst's (and the patient's) subjective experience. This approach invites both participants to enter a field containing the "dialectical" tensions of grappling with and mutually recognizing the other's realities while maintaining their own.

From this frame of reference, the process of "working through" does not place by a post hoc analysis of enactment; rather the working through occurs as patient and analyst "live it together" as an affectively honest intersubjective experience. Unconscious conflict is not ignored in place of an assumed authenticity in the analyst's efforts to be "open." Rather both patient and analyst can consider that which is unconscious from the shared experience of what the enactments call forth into awareness and language.

Analytic outcome, and sometimes the very survival of the treatment, depends on a relational process of working through in which enactment is accepted as giving voice to unconscious and dissociated content. This thinking expands on other contemporary views and emphasizes the relationship be-

Holly Levenkron, L.I.C.S.W., is Codirector, faculty member, and supervising analyst at the Institute of Contemporary Psychotherapy (ICP) in New York City. She is also a faculty member at the Massachusetts Institute of Psychoanalysis (MIP).

tween dissociation, voice, and enactment. It is argued that if this process takes place with sufficient good faith and mutual recognition, each partner's subjective (conscious, unconscious, and dissociated) agenda can become recognizable and, ultimately, "thinkable and speakable" by the other and can provide a fuller range of subjective content for deepening the analytic work.

I offer the view that the analyst's use of self-disclosure is as negotiable as every other part of the patient–analyst relationship and that its clinical value exists only in relation to the level of "affective honesty" that provides its context at a given time.

I'M WRITING ABOUT THE PHENOMENA OF ENACTMENT AND intersubjectivity in clinical practice. Whatever else might be said about these somewhat ambiguous terms, to me in their basic forms they qualify as an unplanned engagement between two subjectivities, creating and negotiating together a unique channel of human communication without which psychoanalysis would not be possible. I chose to call this unique channel the domain of intersubjective space.[1] Yet, as I believe that intersubjective space is a construct that two people can achieve through a collision of their realities (Bromberg, 1996), each person has to surrender "some" of the hold each has on her own subjectivity in order to pay attention to the other, even if that other's view is opposed to her own (as it has to be, simply because it's different).

One important aspect of this experience is that as we try to affect one another, we are also simultaneously being shaped through these efforts. Willingness to let this happen is an inherent part of negotiation, but it isn't about winning; it's about changing our experience to get closer to what we want, while staying related to the other person. To whatever degree we give up our tight hold on our own subjectivity, we increase the potential to validate the other person's subjectivity, while retaining our own. As we are doing this, the experience of relatedness with the other person increases, as can the experiences of learning and of loving. Arriving at any change in relatedness prompts us to continue negotiating (Pizer, 1992) what we want from each other, and after all, isn't what we want from each other, consciously and unconsciously, what motivates enactments and relationship in the first

---

[1]I see intersubjectivity as both a relational field theory (Stolorow, Atwood, and Ross, 1978) and as a developmental achievement theory (Benjamin, 1988). I use the term both ways. In this article my primary usage represents the latter (i.e., a clinical situation that addresses a developmental advance in human relatedness).

place? The flexibility in negotiating this "desire," in whatever form it occurs, is what opens up the enactments and keeps them fluid.

In this essay I do not want to question the quality, perimeters, or ubiquitous nature of enactments. What is more interesting to me is defining the
clinical relationship of enactment to intersubjectivity (Renik, 1997) and negotiating within these dialectic tensions. I am focusing on the process
wherein negotiating enactments becomes "intersubjective relating." I will
depict the evolution of a treatment in which intensely personal affective engagement was the most conspicuous and, arguably, the most clinically
powerful dimension of the analytic process. What I wish to stress is that it is
powerful not as affective honesty per se but as something that can cause the
other person to experience different aspects of what is dissociated or is in
conflict, forcing each person to bring something new—perhaps something
opposite—into mind.

It is important to note that these movements typically take place at lower
intensity than in my work with my patient Ali and are easily disavowed, analyzed away, or considered by many to be "noise" in an otherwise "good"
working alliance. I have selected this case specifically because it places
into *high relief* an openness to the demands of mutual surprise in the psychoanalytic exchange (Stern, 1990). My intention is to provide a close look
at the mutual internal and external progressions between patient and analyst, along with my own sense of moving with this surprise.

During the evolution of every treatment, each person tries to change
the other in terms of her own conscious and unconscious agendas; and to
one degree or another, the need to change the other is often opposed by
that other and often fails as an effort (Slavin and Kriegman, 1998). The
analytic challenge is to allow change in oneself, that is, to allow for the
possibility of the interaction shaping the analyst as well. I have come to
believe that analytic outcome, and sometimes the very survival of the
treatment, depends on whether the process of intersubjective negotiation
takes place with enough good faith that each individual's separate agenda
can become recognizable and ultimately "thinkable" by the other, so that
change in each is facilitated. But what does this mean in terms of psychoanalytic movement?

In the case presented here, my emphasis is on showing how, through
various modes of expression unique to each individual, we (the patient
and I) inevitably pushed against each other's realities from within enactments between us; and, whether we liked it or not, patient and analyst (as
would any two members of a couple) continued to pursue their separate

agendas, both directly and in subtle ways, until each reached a point where something shifted and previous beliefs concerning the way we each had conceptualized the other began to undergo reintegration from within the intersubjective field.

It bears repeating, then, that it is not affective involvement by the analyst per se that creates the therapeutic action. Certainly many others have written about this at length, in particular Darlene Ehrenberg (1984, 1992); Charles Spezanno (1993); Philip Bromberg (1994, 1996); Karen Maroda (1995); and Owen Renik (1996). My particular point is that enactment touches a core element by which something central in the organization of conflict, something that is being denied or dissociated by either party, can be acknowledged and repaired—a process that relies on enactment. Obviously this is more likely in an environment that is both safe enough and provocative enough to invite the expansion of certain agendas along with a sense of self-agency into the interaction (Slavin and Pollack, 1997). I return to this theme throughout.

The clinical craft however, and as I understand it as a tenet of relational work, lies in contacting a part of ourselves through which we can eventually own and reflect on either nonverbally or aloud to our patients what we have discovered about our own participation from within these interactions. This aspect of negotiation makes disclosure as "negotiable" as any other aspect of our communications. Weaving this understanding into the interaction requires that we grapple with an "unresolvable" paradox—the paradox of recognizing the other person's point of view while maintaining our own. It pushes us toward a shift in our behavior to develop a safe space for internal perspectives about ourselves and the other person.

I begin with talking about my treatment of Ali. We had eventually, after several years, reached a point of exhaustion where as she said, "things just weren't working." As we became able to grasp this as a shared experience, the communication process slowly opened and we were able to construct a form of discussion in which the use of confrontation and disclosure moved from enacted power operations to intersubjective relating. This took some time as we both had to find ways to appeal to the other's abilities to listen and change. New kinds of confrontation and disclosure, both loving and adversarial, evolved out of the difficult way we had been communicating; joint decisions about ourselves and our work became possible. As a result, the analytic space became increasingly safe; that is, the relationship became a secure place in which we could explore our connection and examine what was standing in the way of its evolution.

The Analyst's and the Patient's Desire

Ali is a forty-six-year-old woman whom I had been seeing in psychoanalysis three times a week for a number of years. A professional with a doctoral degree in sociology, she came into treatment to overcome debilitating bouts of jealousy coupled with intense feelings of disappointment in a succession of failed relationships with men. Although she had achieved a position of status at the university where she taught and did research, Ali suffered from low self-esteem, considering herself an underachiever. Key relationship patterns in her family included protracted jealousy and anguish in relation to her two more attractive sisters, one of whom had won most of their father's attention. Ali had to contend with this amid her own oppositional and contentious relationship with her father whose love she courted by trying to be more of a peer than a daughter. In opposition to her "feminine" sister and in accord with her father's wish for a son, Ali became athletic, even handsome, in her more masculine style of casual dress and expert at banter and argument. By these means Ali succeeded in engaging her father, but eventually their banter would turn to argument, angering him to the point where dismissing and scornful interactions would erupt, leaving Ali feeling unattractive, unrecognized, and rejected—a loser in the shadow of her two more feminine sisters. She found solace in her relationship with her mother, who, seeming to recognize Ali's style of not fitting, co-opted her daughter into a tight, merged, implicit pact to mutually provide love, safety, and companionship for each other. At first meeting, Ali impressed me as a smart, friendly, insightful, but controlling and aggressive woman with a strong sense of entitlement, which she used to compensate for deep feelings of deprivation, loss, and envy. I will begin with one of many intense encounters.

About one year into our work and shortly before our appointment time, Ali and I had run into each other in my lobby. The elevator was broken and we both headed for the stairs. She held the door and I went first. At one point I turned around and believed I saw her staring at my legs as she climbed behind me. I stopped at the next landing, feeling very uncomfortable. She proceeded past me, continued ahead, and waited for me outside my office. I apologized for the inconvenience of the broken elevator, and we went inside.

Taking her position on the couch she began in a suspended voice, saying almost dazedly, "Well, it was actually OK. It gave me a chance to look at your legs as you climbed the stairs ahead of me." "What are you saying?" I asked, surprised by her candor and intimacy. "Well, I guess I'm saying that it aroused me—sexually. It's just that you have such great legs. You know that, Holly!" She added in an assertive tone, "And I'm sure you know people love to look at them; so I was looking, and it was very nice." Saying this, her voice escalated to shrillness.

Feeling a rush of adrenaline, an uncomfortable tension overtook me. I was repelled at the insinuation that I had shown her a part of my body with the intent to arouse her. I was stunned and unable to speak. She went on, "Holly, you know you like it when someone looks at your legs." This confirmed what had stunned me. It was her direct assumption that I had just consented to having some form of sex with her, that I had choreographed the maneuver. In a strong tone that carried the ring of a question, I said, "I find it hard to believe that you really think I would do that to arouse you."

She said, again mockingly, "Well, you did walk ahead of me. You knew I would look at your legs. Now, now, Holly." She was shaking her index finger at me from the couch as if to say "Now, now—you bad girl." Our experiences of this event were clearly very different. Knowing this, however, did not stop me from wondering to myself how she had the nerve to speak to me with this kind of familiarity; that is, knowing this did not stop me from wondering how she was having this experience.

The confusion was simple: here, in this aspect of herself, she felt foreign to me, and this feeling was frightening. She was exhibiting a belief that we had shared a certain kind of intimacy that was not predicated on anything I was aware of. Knowing this, I still didn't know what to say to her. I was numb and became passive in the throes of her aggressive overtures. I felt so bad, so confused that I began to consider whether I did want her to notice my legs and whether it gave me a certain kind of narcissistic pleasure to walk up the stairs in front of her. Was I, in fact, aroused? Then I came to what I thought were my senses. I realized that any natural desire I had to be admired, along with my ability to feel flattered if someone gave me a compliment, was perfectly all right. Only now that natural desire had been transformed into self-repudiating dread, a dread that made my own desire to be a playful and flirtatious person seem dirty. Consequently I couldn't speak to her from a playful and flirtatious self that could both enjoy and accept her sexuality (Knoblauch, 1997). It was a no-win situation, and I found myself pulling back, withdrawing, and getting agitated. We both had to be deprived.

In this instance we were both shaping the other. In his modification of traditional self psychological theory, Morrison talks about the way we attempt to shape each other (and invite being given shape by the other to provide for specific needs). This "cocreated" selfobject often provides a better experience than the one inherent in the environment. In this case, however, Ali was assuming a relationship I was not offering. Given the manner she was asking for something, I had, in the language of self psychology; that is, I had to fail to provide her selfobject needs at this point—if for no other reason than I couldn't—didn't want to—meet them. I didn't want to be the person whom she was making me out to be. I learned, on the other hand, that I could offer her something else that might allow or encourage her to reshape her ideal of what kind of selfobject experience I could or would provide. The relational challenge for me was, how could I do this reshaping in the storm of my countertransference, and how could Ali participate in this reshaping in the storm of her transference strivings? The relational, or mutual failings—wherein we both had to be deprived—took the form of Ali's failing to get anything from me because of her distancing and assuming behavior, and my failing to take pleasure, the pleasure commonly derived from liking another; my own protective defenses prevented me from reaching out to her in a loving way. Unless one of us shifted, we would have to remain here for a while.

I experienced her expressions as "I need you to desire me—I need to have a certain significance to you that requires you to put aside your own self—your own subjectivity." But for me to desire her, or anyone, I could not accept the requirement to put aside my subjectivity, and shouldn't have to. She was hurt because, although there was an erotic component to her desire, what she wanted from me was more complicated. I later came to see it was about her wish and fantasy that I desire her to desire me. This was conveyed to me in her remark "C'mon Holly, you wanted me to look at your legs and you know it!"

As time went on, my transference became fairly vivid. Specifically, I felt Ali consistently attempting to force my hand to get what she wanted. Consequently I became stifled and more defended. Certainly part of her anger was caused by the deprivation she experienced from my stifled emotions. At first, in this defended place, I dissociated my ability to regulate how much I could take in without feeling assaulted. Regulating this included finding a way to express, without alienating her, that I didn't like what she was doing to me. I understood the pattern to be that whenever she became desirous her transference repetitions led her to revert to a self that bore resemblance to the "little tyke" who battled wits with her critical, alcoholic father. I gathered that that voice enabled her to dissociate her longing for tenderness, while maintaining the excitement that permitted her to feel safer in the shadow of her father's power. Thus, as a defense against certain longings, her teasing aggression must have become relationally satisfying. In this voice, her loving and erotic feelings were preserved and protected although rarely satisfied.

Although we spoke often and in a variety of ways about these constellations, such apparently mutative discussions occurred during more vulnerable affective states when certain transference "beliefs" were active. For example, her demand that we experience the "ecstasy of at-one-ment," to use Tustin's apt developmental phrase cited by Mitrani (1998, p.102), combined the aggressive stance she took with her father and the merger she experienced with her mother. This seemed a lethal combination in relationships, and it felt impossible for me to meet. Nothing I tried up to then had seemed to loosen this knot. Although unhappy with my responses, I remained angry at her refusal to release me and let our relationship develop in a more natural way. From within the experience of these tensions, I recall feeling very bad—being quite troubled—for wanting to reject Ali. This bad feeling gnawed at me because despite my powerful concern to speak to her, I didn't want to hurt her feelings. Yet, I couldn't imagine telling her what it was that so fiercely stopped me from being able to love her. Being stuck between my own boundaries and Ali's pain was very uncomfortable. It was here that something had to shift.

Returning here to the session, I recall getting lost in my own thoughts about this dilemma. I found myself associating to remembered incidents of her childhood, in particular her involvement with her friend's boyfriend at age seventeen and periods of minor shoplifting at about age twenty. From the confluence of my feelings and experiences of failure, having tried more traditional efforts to analyze her aggression and envy, I saw the necessity of changing my approach. I felt it made sense for me to say something more direct—an effort to connect my experience to hers. I said, "You know, I know it's been hard for you, but I wonder if you believe you'll never get anything unless you take it. So you don't wait until it's offered and instead go right for it?" I paused, her silence stirring a desire in me to make this more personal. I added, still in a strong tone, "The problem is, you can't really get it like that—love just doesn't work that way. I can't give it to you just because you want it. But I will give it to you if I want to—you just have to let me do that in my own time." I felt this was an honest expression of a significant difficulty. Because she wanted so much from me, she was blinded to the reality that I had to decide these things for myself. Ali later told me how she experienced this as a powerful and meaningful communication. She started to cry, and I felt shaken.

While I was able to locate my difficulty in giving her what she wanted when she demanded it from me and, further, was able to tell her something about what I needed to become more intimate with her, which in itself held her through her anger because it explicitly stated a desire to continue a relationship with her, I was not yet able to address the shame that underlay her contempt for me. After all of this, Ali said, "Now I feel as if you're going to leave me." I heard this as her attempt, using herself as agent, to participate in the negotiation. Whether or not it was a demand, for some reason I didn't hear it as demanding. I responded, "I'm here, I'm not going anywhere. But you can push me away if you insist I give you all of me." This was extremely calming for her. Although it included an honest expression of my anger, which frightened her, it also expressed my attachment and commitment to her as well as her capacity to have an impact on me. She could infer that I was both concerned about and willing to communicate about what I saw as a problem and that I believed it was critical for both of us to consider this as part of improving our relationship. In this frame she could hear it. My comment was regulating, showing that I recognized her as an important participant in our relationship.

These statements, which were rather direct, would not have had a chance at being heard if they did not contain, implicitly, a compassionate element, letting her know that I could indeed envision giving her something, only she wasn't giving me the chance. I had to ask myself, however, if I felt she could be touched by compassion. I didn't know. If I had tried to explain my observations to her—to formalize them into a statement or interpretation while we were in the throes of the experience—I would have lost her. My explanation would have been felt as absenting myself from the experience, making this, in Racker's (1968) famous words "an interaction between a sick person and a healthy one" (p. 132). It would not have addressed my acknowledgment of her experience as part of an intersubjective field in which we both had come to polarize each other.

I hope a central way I work can be seen in my attempt to achieve the affective honesty contained in these statements. Such affective honesty becomes a powerful source of therapeutic action because of its power to communicate my own conscious and unconscious agenda, as well as providing a background in which my patient could experience her own impact on me. However, I believe the effectiveness of this type of communication depends on the analyst's not insisting that the patient adopt the analyst's point of view. In this context, in my work with Ali, my affect contained and conveyed to Ali feelings of both anger and a wish for connection. It shaped the communication to Ali that I felt deprived of an important experience with her, telling her what I needed in order to maximize the opportunity for her to get what she wanted and for me to get what I wanted. Since she had the choice to consider this implicit and explicit request, her sense of responsibility and self-agency were elicited.

I've implied that in an intersubjective field, our actions are motivated by a confluence of desires associated with things we want and need from each other. This desire may be the primary organizing principle that makes us "prewired" to strive for relationship, and it may be the charge that keeps enactments fertile. The point is that patient and analyst both struggle, internally and interpersonally, with their separate needs to be recognized or desired. Eros, the fundamental marker of the force of desire, was embedded in Ali's body, in her sexual strivings. Eros, as it encompasses recognition, linked drive with a relational outcome. The intense "physical" representation of Ali's desire embodied, as well as grounded, her wishes to be recognized. Until the interpersonal field could shift, so that we could negotiate the experience of her erotic–aggressive feelings in the relational context in which they were situated (Dimen, 1995), these feelings remained a looming presence between us.

Dissociation and Enactment: A Dialectic

On one particular Friday I came into my office feeling rather bleak. I had been through a week of serious decision making with my husband in regard to ending our seventeen-year marriage. Generally upbeat and playful, I was simply exhausted and looked it, but nevertheless felt that I could see that day's patients. I decided to take a week off to contemplate a final decision beginning the next day. Yet, despite my sense that I could see my patients that day I was definitely not myself, and I may not have realized how much I needed from others. Announcing to Ali that I was taking a week-long break, apologizing for the short notice, I said something personal had happened that had to be dealt with. Having done this all that day to mixed reviews, I thought I was prepared for any reaction.

She was very upset, although curious, and she grilled me about what it was that would take me away so suddenly. What was so striking and unusual about her reaction were her fantasies of all the "wonderful" things about to happen to me. I was getting upset as she got in touch with the aspect of herself that, when insecure and envious, becomes filled with rage and is blinded to any prior recognition—something we had experienced many times before. I could see it coming, perhaps with my mind's eye, but it was fairly palpable. Aware of a shift, I noticed her body go limp, and she folded her hands on her stomach. Turning her face to the wall and saying a few sentences that were tangential, she spoke in a slow, halted, breathy voice. I was getting angry, but I was not aware of it at this point. She breathed deeply. When she got like this, her voice took on a controlled, condescending tone. I found it hard to concentrate. It was as if the room was filling up with an uncomfortable chemical—perhaps the projection of adrenaline. As with adrenaline, it worked as a signal to prepare for attack. Did I want to placate her, to soothe her? No. At that moment I wanted it out on the table where I could see it. After a while, I told her I was experiencing her envy as overwhelming, that although she did not actually know why I was leaving, she assumes everything in my life is good. "Yes," she said—pausing—"I am very mad!" Packing anger and envy, she shot the following words my way: "I can't stand the way you talk to me! You are so fucking mean! Who do you think you are, Holly? No one talks to me that way, only you! You're sorry for the short notice. Well, what about me?" It was out on the table.

Any mention of my life collided with Ali's envy, causing a shift to her feeling that she had nothing and would remain having nothing. From what seemed this aspect of herself and with the same pained, hungry familiarity I mentioned earlier—as if we were a couple who were having a fight—she dramatically listed what she thought I'd be doing on my week off. "So, Holly, you're going away with your husband and you didn't want to tell me. What did you want to hide? Huh? Holly? Sneaking off to some beautiful summer house where you have nice friends, maybe a pool. Have a nice time with your husband. Just the two of you. Nice Holly—cozy—go ahead. I'll stay here in the hot city. You go have fun." It went on. I had difficulty holding onto my composure and found myself unable to listen. With tears welling in my eyes, which I suspected she couldn't see, I tried as hard as I could to refrain from telling her exactly what had happened to me that week. I was in touch with a strong wish for her to stop torturing me. At this moment, I was sick of the god-awful envy that turned this intelligent, professional, sometimes caring woman into a monster—envy that we were no closer to understanding and alleviating.

After some time of her unstoppable poking at me, I found myself struggling with a powerful urge to tell her every bad thing that had ever happened to me; that is, I wanted to tell her just how hard my life had really been and how hard it certainly was at this time. I also wanted to tell her to shut up. I couldn't remove myself from the explosions going off inside of me to gain the distance I needed to speak to her in a calm way. Yet I didn't tell her anything about my personal situation. I knew I had to stop her ranting, for my sake and for hers. In an angry tone I asserted, "Look, I won't be responsible for what you didn't get, only for what I don't give you, and right now this is all I can give you. Next week that may change." At this moment it didn't matter what I said; just being me was enough for her to be in an envious rage. It meant I was separate.

Nondisclosure as a Substitution for Confrontation

In not telling her what had happened, that my marriage was breaking up, I thought I was protecting her from feeling guilty for attacking me. I was also avoiding what I imagined to be a sadistic retort from her, which would confirm what I experienced as her fantasy of ownership over me. I imagined her reaction would be "Great, Holly, now we're in the same boat." And we were. We were both experiencing broken agreements. Over the next few weeks I was steadfast in my belief that telling her would be relational suicide, that I'd be doing this just to give her what she wanted, to calm her down or to carry out my illusion that she would feel remorse for her actions. At that time, I could not formulate (Stern, 1983) the pull I fought against to tell all, as when the emotional and articulated demands of the patient to intrude into the therapist's privacy are so great that she has to tell—for the wrong reasons. To her, telling was a way to cement a bond of love. I felt it was a way of cementing a bond of enslavement.

Although nondisclosure here was a clear expression of my subjectivity (Aron, 1996), I am not advancing a "technical mandate" of nondisclosure. In fact, typically not subscribing to the use of disclosure in a prescribed way, believing, as I discussed earlier, that disclosure can be negotiated from within the mutual exchanges between patient and analyst, I will later address how I approached it quite differently at another point in the work (Ehrenberg, 1995; Greenberg, 1995; Renik, 1995, 1996; Mitchell, 1998). Along with many others, my manner is consistent with my belief that therapeutic action often depends on disclosure of the analyst's experience of the patient (Bromberg, 1994; Ehrenberg, 1995; Renik, 1995, 1996). Here, however, I used nondisclosure as a foil to avoid abuse of my privacy and admission of my vulnerability. In my withdrawal and silence, I was unaware of how I was enacting my self-protection and my right to privacy. I dissociated my ability to voice my boundaries—to talk to her about why I could not talk to her. Convinced I understood what was going on, I avoided any internal cues that would have taken me closer to negotiating differently. Albeit about dissociation, this example fundamentally links disclosure to the aims of the relational experience (conscious or unconscious) that provide the context for it. This idea returns to what I had addressed earlier; that is, self-disclosure is as negotiable, or nonnegotiable, as every other aspect of the patient–analyst relationship.

Affective Honesty

The "realness" of an interaction is significant as a metaphor or channel for the analyst's honest expression. Its value is not only in its recognition of being authentic but in its implied offer to the patient of the opportunity to reorganize fantasies and projections about the analyst that help the patient establish what is going on inside the analyst's mind (Fonagy, 1991). While there is importance in analyzing fantasies some of the time, at other times "revealing" the analyst's thoughts is often a relief to the patient, even if it opens up rage and painful feelings, because it makes things clear. The inclusion of the analyst's "realness," whether in terms of conflict, affect, or agenda, has been advanced in the writings of many analysts including Bird (1972); Ehrenberg (1974, 1984); Greenberg (1991); Frankel (1993); Spezzano (1993); Renik (1993b, 1996); Bromberg (1994,1996); Davies (1994); Maroda (1995); Aron (1996, 1998); Slavin and Pollack (1997); Mitchell (1998); and Slavin and Kriegman (1998). One thing that I have been interested in and hope I have learned through these exchanges is that "being real" and connecting with another person cannot always occur through loving gestures. My approach with this patient was generally aimed at enlisting our relationship, and accepting this idea presented me with an interpersonal challenge calling for a dramatic shift. I wanted to strike a balance between protecting her (recognizing her vulnerability) and protecting myself so that her subjectivity did not do violence to me, while at the same time maintaining an open channel to express my point of view. I found this task to be conflictual and it became a focus of my own growth.

What I came to understand was that to have my own voice was not synonymous with aggression. Essentially, I became able to say to my patient, "I'm not going to let your subjectivity destroy mine, nor should I, because then I wouldn't exist (and vice versa)." Here I was regulating my ability to tolerate assault—something I had difficulty doing earlier. The key of this regulation is to know that we don't have to agree with each other's reality, nor in the therapeutic exchange do we even have to convince the other person to agree with us. The analytic stance here is for both of us to recognize that we have different realities (Ehrenberg, 1985; Benjamin, 1988; Bromberg, 1991a,b, 1998; Renik, 1993a, 1998), and the negotiation lies in developing the freedom to tell each other our experiences of it. I would have to learn to do this or I would be stuck along with Ali in this place of mutual annihilation.

Figuring out ways to move out of power plays, however subtle, opened up the experience of connection and safety for both of us. As is probably evident, however, Ali and I had a fit that supplied us with endless opportunities for stepping into particular types of power plays. For Ali, envy was a disintegrated product of my separateness. She hated my life and everything in it because it made me separate. I had unconsciously opted to dissociate that part of myself that could experience her shame and negotiate this envy and instead often entered into power plays with her. That is, while I could find expression for my anger, an anger that was understandable, it was an irresponsible anger because I couldn't confront her with it in an integrated way. This type of expression of my anger did not lend itself to productive exploration and was not satisfying for either of us as an analytic way of life. Just as intersubjective relating is not synonymous with expression of agreement or merger, asserting oneself as a separate subject is not synonymous with any and all forms of expression. My recognizing a colliding of our agendas (I wanted freedom where merger was threatening; she wanted merger where freedom was threatening) was an important turning point in shifting my direction (Bromberg, 1996; Harris, 1996). Two subjects wanting what were actually diverging agendas was not the most problematic issue; getting polarized in these wants was what foreclosed relatedness. I was intensely aware that I was not relating to my patient. It is not by establishing relatedness that we open up communication; it is the opening up of communication that establishes relatedness. We were having ongoing experiences that kept the focus of the treatment too tightly held on her relationship with me. As I was clearly getting caught up in power plays myself, I began to wonder if I wasn't able to let go. Once I started thinking this way I was able to explore speaking to her without the intent of being understood—just with the wish of being considered (Renik, 1993a). This permitted a different kind of confrontation that freed me from some of my own control operations.

Confrontation and Intersubjectivity

The awareness that we didn't like certain things about each other, made clear by our efforts to articulate our thoughts, put Ali and me at risk. Articulating can test connections by making explicit heretofore unknown things that had maintained their shape only in fantasy. I found we were also able to communicate this risk to our connection, however, which helped immeasurably. At some point, my message shifted to "You know I don't agree with you, but I could feel closer to you if you stopped trying to control me and tried to see more of who I am; that is, that you see me less as a transference figure and more as a complex person who sometimes looks like your parents and at other times can be someone new." Her stance shifted too and began to resemble something like "I find it hard to believe I could trust you. I prefer to see you as a controlling monster (father), but that is clearly not getting me anywhere and I'm getting tired." The following session elaborates this type of affectively real confrontation and how it works with both patient and analyst.

Session Three

Ali was going on vacation, and typically separations were upsetting. In fact, early in the treatment we had done a considerable amount of work around break points. On this occasion, she hesitated at the door before leaving to tell me something. She looked sad when she said, "I hope you'll be all right." Although we were already at the door, I inquired about this. I was well aware of the separation that took place about a year and a half before when I went into the hospital for a congenital aortic valve replacement surgery. Although Ali and I had experienced other separations since then, such as her vacations and mine, I felt concerned about her fears. "What is it?" I asked. "Well, I'm worried you may get sick—your heart." Because of the reality of the past surgery, I reassured her that there was nothing wrong with me, I went on to reiterate that this had had to be corrected sooner or later, that it just turned out to be sooner. I have a normal heart otherwise, I told her. In fact, now my heart is better than before. We both smiled. I said,

"Really, I'm fine." One week later she returned. I sat down and she grinned in a familiar, penetrating way. "So! You survived my absence, Holly? You didn't die without me!"

I answered with a serious question, "Is your grin telling me something?" I felt an old sense of constriction and a wish to back away, only I wanted to stay connected to the good feeling I experienced with her when she left. She said nothing. I waited a while and then finally asked directly, "Did you want to hear that I couldn't live without you?"

"Yes, that's true. I wanted you to miss me, to hold me in your thoughts the way I think about you. To think about me all the time, and wish I were here. I was upset when I left! You didn't seem to care enough." She went on with how she didn't know if she were getting anywhere in therapy; she was tired of coming, it was so long. Maybe she should stop. I told her I didn't experience it like that at all. Even though the subject of my surgery was real, adding to the tensions of separations for Ali, I did start to get angry. I was aware that I also felt threatened. No one likes to hear that someone is thinking about leaving, especially when it feels manipulative. She hadn't acted this way for some time, though, and I didn't know why this was happening now. All I knew was that she was escalating things, using an issue that could have brought us closer to separate us; she had missed me and was worried. Perhaps I felt that, regardless of the emotions stirred by the surgery and her awareness that I was mortal, I couldn't attend to a reunion between us if she was dismissing the other good aspects in our relationship. I decided to address what was standing in my way.

"What is going on?" I asked. "You may think I know—but I don't!" "Nothing," she said, "But you can't take my having strong feelings." I responded, "I think I can take it. But look, Ali, I'd like to say what's on my mind—which is that I just don't agree with you. You come in and tell me you want me to keep you in my thoughts and think highly of you. Well I do. I like you, I care about you, and I do think highly of you. I've been telling you that for some time. So, what is this? No, I think it is about your wanting me to need you so much that I would not be able to tolerate your absence— to have you in my every thought. Even more so, you want me to tell you that. But I can't do that, and, what's more, I shouldn't have to. Especially under threat of siege. And if I don't act a certain way, then you lose out on anything else I do give you."

"Yes. It's true," she said with a little reflection, and I believed she meant it. I told her that I didn't feel that what she was showing me or the way she went about trying to get something from me was love or even close to it. I thought it was a wish—a demand—for me to love her. I wanted to have a loving feeling for her, I told her, but she was suffocating me by demanding it. I said (here I stopped myself from hesitating), "Ali, look, this could destroy this therapy, this relationship. I don't want that to happen. So help me out here." She stayed with me, saying, "I don't know what you mean by destroy. I know you're talking about some sort of need I have to merge with you—I do—and I get blinded by it. The thought that popped into my head was about something I felt years ago when I had the fantasy of being inside of you. I used to think about it a lot but it hasn't been present for years." I told her my experience was that it has been present for a long time. I was referring to a memory of the intensity of her intermittent dazed states. She looked puzzled. "When?" "Well," I said, "in the years that we have struggled with your envy of me. With my separateness." She looked alert and asked, "Is that why you said it was destructive?"

I answered by saying that I thought so, but that I didn't know, adding "Do you feel that my being separate means you would be alone forever?"

She answered, "I would rather be inside of you and connected that way than to face the world alone. Lately I have been thinking about leaving therapy—that it has been a long time and I've grown a lot. I don't know what else I can do, but then I get scared and think that I'll never be able to leave, that I have to stay, and I get depressed that my fears can never end."

I said, "This feels more honest to me." I felt a shift and added, "I don't think anyone ever showed you that you can be safe even if you are separate. I think your mother showed you the opposite."

When I asked her if my going in for surgery had left her feeling that I would die and leave her unprotected, she began to cry. At this point in the session I was able to tell her that I hadn't realized how frightening that must have been for her, but this time as she left for vacation I did realize it. I said that I was sorry for not understanding how scared she was of losing me. We had not talked this openly before. Something had shifted, and I was aware of wanting to act on my interest to be more open. I told her that I was OK, but of course we would all die. No one had ever told her before, I reflected, that she would be OK if it happened to someone she was connected with. Her job all her life was to make sure her mother was emotionally taken care of. Then, just as I was speaking to Ali I had the strangest memory. I recalled that as my mother was dying, she would not let me cry; furthermore, she did not even consider that I needed to be protected in any way. She just denied her own death and wouldn't let me in on it. I was terrified, and later when I saw that I could survive her death, I wished I could have shared more with her. With this memory in my thoughts, I asked Ali if it were possible during the last leg of our work together to include our considering that I will die at some point, even if I didn't die for a while, and that she would be OK. After all I told her, even though we are about the same age, no one knows when they will die. She cried and said she didn't believe she could ever take that in or bear that. I told her I believed she could. I wasn't sure where this was taking us, but it felt crucial, honest, and related.

Associating to the beginning of the session Ali said she had a strange bodily experience, similar to the ones she had earlier in treatment when she would occasionally get scared and perceive herself to be floating away. Once, when she had expressed acute fear at this feeling, I told her the couch would hold her. She was enormously relieved by my response then, as if she had feared she had become disconnected, dissociated. We had never quite understood these bodily experiences that had returned as we were discussing death and separation. It was as if she were enacting something with her body—speaking to me through it. She started to cry, and said how amazing it was that she had actually achieved a lot in her life and was really basically OK, yet all she wanted to do was to be curled up in my womb. She said that in the last session hearing me talk to her about separation she had actually felt a strong longing to merge into me, physically, as she and I talked. It had frightened her, and she began to feel spacey as if she were floating across the room toward me.

She was able to calm herself and to ask what this feeling was. Although I thought she knew, I suggested it might be a beginning recognition of separation. She said it was frightening and OK. I told her, "No one ever talked to you about being separate, but what is more important for us is that no one ever separated from you in a loving way." The session ended here.

Discussion

I have addressed the analytic relationship as an "alive" experience between two people who try over a range of efforts, both subtle and direct, conscious and unconscious, to get their individual needs met. In all situations of "relationship", I believe, this is a basic human striving. I argue that for analytic treatment to be successful, we must depend on the continuing negotiation of this fundamental interpersonal activity, the activity, that is, of getting the object of our desire, more specifically, getting the object of our desire to recognize us. This central idea sets up a field containing the failsafe of desiring to preserve the relationship. However, this same desire fills us with expectations that we strive for, often, as can be seen with Ali, in ways that prevent this very desire from being realized.

These relational strivings determine the course of our precisely differing agendas and render enactment ever-present. Yet, I believe it is this precise desire that is at the heart of therapeutic action, with therapeutic action rooted in the analyst's ability to engage her desire, to "invite" the patient to negotiate, with safety, particular stuck points.

Enactment and Dissociation

I argue that the working through of transferential enactments is not accomplished afterwards by a post hoc analysis but from within the aliveness of the experience, as part of what patient and analyst live through together. Even with contemporary acceptance of enactment as a routine part of human behavior, it is still often discussed as something that "happens" out of the ordinary course of treatment, a thing that is accepted as long as it is analyzed later. The problem in this idea is that "enacted" experiences are separated from other forms of mental process, making their analysis a separate order of thinking removed from the aliveness of the experience.

I believe my work with Ali would not have developed to a full analytic end if I had proceeded as though enactments are pathological, delimited entities that required fixing in time and are only later analyzed through interpretation. Along with many others, I emphasize that enactment exists at all times as the substrate of analytic interaction (Wolstein, 1959; Levenson, 1983; Ehrenberg, 1992; Renik, 1993b; Aron, 1996). Renik's (1997) radical usage specifies that "there is only enactment (singular), a constant, unavoidable aspect of everything patient and analyst do in analysis" (p. 282). This assertion underscores my own working definition of enactment, which is an unplanned, ongoing engagement representing the very nature of mental process, choreographed moment to moment as we associate and dissociate (Davies, 1998) to another person's conscious and unconscious fantasies. This self- and field-regulating behavior (Mitchell, 1988), seen in a mutual act, explains enactments as being constructed around both the dissociated *and* conscious aspects (fantasies) of both parties. As these aspects are intricately connected, the analytic advantage for their expansion is that they hold the potential for expression of both. The key issue here, whether or not we agree that enactment is always occurring, is how one defines and uses clini-

cally the coming into conscious awareness the phenomenon called enactment, because it is only here in awareness that we can consciously act on it.

Confrontation and Intersubjectivity

An essential component of mutuality is that of making the awareness of
separate realities a foundation for all negotiations. However, I argue for a
form of therapeutic action that is based on a type of confrontation, one that
becomes intersubjective when it addresses what Benjamin refers to as the
fundamental paradox of recognition, which she states as, "a constant tension between recognizing the other and asserting the self" (Benjamin,
1992, p. 51). That is, when the analyst can state his point of view by offering his "experience" of the patient, as long as he does not insist that the patient give up his sense of reality (Ehrenberg, 1984; Bromberg, 1991b, 1998;
Renik, 1993a, 1998; Mitchell, 1997).

Winnicott (1969b) describes the importance of confrontation in regard
to what he called the "adolescent challenge" (p. 147). He writes "The word
confrontation is used here to mean that a grown-up person stands up and
claims the right to have a personal point of view " (p. 147, italics mine). Although he doesn't use the term, Winnicott lays the foundation for an
intersubjective theory of relating when he states that the infant, to become a
subject in his own right, first has to recognize the mother as a subject. To do
this the infant has to experience the destruction of the "mother as object" in
order to recreate–relocate her through his own subjective experience of her
survival (Winnicott, 1969a). One way of reading Winnicott incorporates
this achievement as representing a "one-person" experience, not yet
intersubjective. It mandates a loving, selfless other to meet the child's aggressive acts, and thus prescribes as technique (Greenberg, 1991) the style
of survival the mother is to take. This schema becomes relational
(intersubjective) with a different reading of Winnicott, when the object—
the mother—who survives as a subject can be recognized by the child over
a range of affective exchanges (Benjamin, 1992).

Affectively "Real" Confrontation

Whether loving or adversarial, as part of the trajectory of relatedness confrontation plays an important role in the coming into awareness of previ-

ously dissociated content, not through insight gained from the "wisdom" in the confrontation but from what the confrontation calls up for our consideration. Confrontations make people work, not because they are threatening but because they touch on biases that have prevented us from making use of new perspectives. In accord with the many analysts who have written on the value of confrontation and inclusion of "real" feelings (including Winnicott, 1969b; Bird, 1972; Ehrenberg, 1974, 1992; Frankel, 1993; Renik, 1993b, 1996; Davies, 1994; Bromberg, 1995, 1996; Slavin and Pollack, 1997), I believe the analyst must be willing to put some of her feelings and experiences on the line so that patient and analyst can grapple with the "real" conflict they feel. I'm convinced that if this does not occur, despite our therapeutic advances away from the blank screen model, the therapist still can remain a "bundle of projections" (Winnicott, 1969a, p. 88), and conflict, remaining in effigy, is only incompletely worked through (Freud, 1912). As I stated earlier, inclusion of the analyst's affect is essential to communicate the strength of conviction in the content communicated. Mayer (1996) says it is "the fire of each heart meeting the fire of each mind that makes for the intensity of analytic work" (p. 159). This concept applies whether confrontations are loving or adversarial, but the analyst's ability to do this with the patient must be earned. There were two confrontations illustrated in the second and third sessions, the first in the second session, adversarial, and the next in the third session, loving. In both I emphasized with conviction and compassion my experience of Ali and myself, not my certainty about her reality. One way that I learned to work "affectively" with her was by understanding that confrontation and compassion were both necessary to work with shared emotional experience.

Knowledge and Authority in Therapeutic Action

It goes without saying that questions can and should arise regarding this approach. If the analyst voices his or her opinion, it is possible that the power shifts toward the analyst and unduly influences the patient (Price, 1997). Price cautions against the illusion that we can escape our own ties to power. The distinction between unearned authority (Renik, 1996) and power (Stein, 1997) emphasizes a "positive" form of power in the analytic setting. The continuum of power and authority is available to the most well-intended analyst, making it desirable for the analyst's actions to be accorded conscious, explicit scrutiny (Renik, 1996). Over time, Ali and I discussed our interactions with increasing comfort, partially because the development of candor is a natural evolution arising out of any successful negotiation and partially because we both learned that articulating what we experienced did not lead to irreparable ruptures in attachment.

In this light, mutual disclosure of our thinking becomes collaborative and therefore negotiable, rather than power based. We face an unavoidable relational dilemma if we adopt a stance that encourages us to voice our point of view, unless we are open to hearing about our own blind spots and are able to reconsider our positions, as well as the urgency with whom we present them. Mutative impact, then, is enhanced by recognizing that someone will not change just because we need or want him to. If we can access this awareness we are able to repair with the patient at least some of those moments that could become power plays. This in itself can have a healing effect. At the same time, if we can hold onto our subjectivity in the service of maintaining a separate reality, both analyst and patient can say to the other, "Your subjectivity is not sufficient to neutralize mine. I'm sorry, but that's just the way it is. Certain differences that exist between us may never be resolved, but we can go on and still have a connection, and even love, between us. Although I may not be getting it right or agreeing with you, I can respond honestly from my own experience to the impact I may have on your subjectivity."

When Ali experienced my statements as control operations (which they sometimes were), she could do nothing but fight and shut down her desire to be more related. She would then cling tenaciously to old viewpoints (as did I when I perceived her to be treating me that way). At such times, whether Ali or I were angry, withdrawn, or expressing warm feelings, if these expressions affected the work by keeping the system closed (Ringstrom, 1998), one of us had to attempt to open it. For some time it was my role. Control as a fundamental interpersonal operation is unavoidable. We can't predict how something we experience one way will be viewed by someone else. Because of our separate agendas, control operations are inevitable. They are also a necessary aspect of what is communicated in analysis because a patient can be "cured" by making us aware of our control operations (as the patient experiences them). These control operations will be evoked no matter how hard we try to erase them from our repertoire. In this way our patients make us aware of what we may have dissociated and by the patient's impact on us, through the enactments, we gain the opportunity to give up that control or attempt to alter it. If we don't, because we are entrenched in one thing or another, a patient doesn't grow and neither do we.

Through the enactments and our "affective honesty", we can show patient's their impact on us, offering them a new perspective on us as well as on their own sense of agency. Enactment is basically, after all, the *ongoing* playing out of our wishes and fantasies to change and influence the other in ways of which we are often not aware. I hope I have shown that ideally the process of what we call "working through an enactment" does not take place through post hoc analysis but rather that the working through is the analysis and occurs as we live it. This is the negotiation.

REFERENCES

Aron, L. (1996), *A Meeting of Minds: Mutuality in Psychoanalysis*. Hillsdale, NJ: The Analytic Press.

_____ (1998), Clinical choices and the theory of psychoanalytic technique. *Psychoanal. Dial.* 8:207–216.

Benjamin, J. (1988), *Bonds of Love*. New York: Pantheon.

_____ (1992), Recognition and destruction: An outline of intersubjectivity. In: *Relational Perspectives in Psychoanalysis,* ed. N.J. Skolnick, S.C. Warshaw. Hillsdale, NJ: The Analytic Press, pp.43–60.

Bird, B. (1972), Transference: Universal phenomenon and the hardest part of analysis. *Journal of the American Psychoanalytic Association.* 20:267–301.

Bromberg, P.M. (1991a), On knowing one's patient inside out: The aesthetics of unconscious communication. *Psychoanal. Dial.* 1:899–422.

_____ (1991b), Reply to discussion by Enid Balint, *Psychoanal. Dial.*1:431–437.

_____ (1994), "Speak! That I may see you": Some reflections on dissociation, reality and psychoanalytic listening. *Psychoanal. Dial.* 4:517–548.

_____ (1995), Resistance, object–usage, and human relatedness. *Contemp.Psychoanal.* 31:173–192.

_____ (1996), Standing in the spaces: The multiplicity of self and the psychoanalytic relationship. *Contemp. Psychoanal.* 32:509–536.

_____ (1998), Staying the same while changing: Reflections on clinical judgment. *Psychoanal. Dial.* 8:225–236.

Davies, J.M. (1994), Love in the afternoon: A relational reconsideration of desire and dread in the countertransference. *Psychoanal. Dial.* 4:153–170.

_____ (1998), Multiple perspectives on multiplicity. *Psychoanal. Dial.* 8:195–206.

Dimen, M. (1995), On "our nature": Prolegomenon to a relational theory of sexuality. In: *Disorienting Sexuality: Psychoanalytic Reappraisals of Sexual Identities,* ed. T. Domenici and R.C. Lesser. New York:Routledge. pp. 129–153.

Ehrenberg, D.B. (1974), The intimate edge in therapeutic relatedness. *Contemp. Psychoanal.* 10:423–437.

_____ (1984), Psychoanalytic engagement II: Affective considerations. *Contemp. Psychoanal.* 20:560–581.

_____ (1985), Countertransference resistance. *Contemp. Psychoanal.* 21:563–576.

_____ (1992), *The Intimate Edge,* New York: W.W. Norton & Co.

_____ (1995), Self disclosure: Therapeutic tool or indulgence? *Contemp. Psychoanal.* 31:213–228.

Fonagy, P. (1991), Thinking about thinking: Some clinical and theoretical considerations in the treatment of a borderline patient. *International Journal of Psycho-Analysis,* 72:639–656.

Frankel, J. (1993), Collusion and intimacy in the analytic relationship. In: *The Legacy of Sandor Ferenczi,* ed., L. Aron, and A. Harris. Hillsdale, NJ: The Analytic Press, pp. 227–247.

Freud, S. (1912), The dynamics of transference. *Standard Edition.* 12:99–108. London: Hogarth Press.

Greenberg, J. (1991), Countertransference and reality. *Psychoanal. Dial.* 1:52–73.

_____ (1995), Self disclosure: Is it psychoanalytic? *Contemp. Psychoanal.* 31:193–205.

Harris, A. (1996), The conceptual power of multiplicity. *Contemp. Psychoanal.* 32:537–552.

Knoblauch, S. (1997), The play and interplay of passionate experience: Multiple organizations of desire. *Gender and Psychoanalysis.* 2:323–343.

Levenson, E. (1983), *The Ambiguity of Change.* New York: Basic Books.

_____ (1994), Beyond countertransference: Aspects of the analyst's desire. *Contemp. Psychoanal.* 30:691–707.

Maroda, K. (1995), Show some emotion: Completing the cycle of affective communication. Presented at a meeting of the Division of Psychoanalysis (39), American Psychological Association, Santa Monica, Ca.

Mayer, E.L. (1996), Changes in science and changing ideas about knowledge and authority in psychoanalysis. *Psychoanal. Quart.* 65:158–200.

Mitchell, S.A. (1988), *Relational Concepts in Psychoanalysis: An Integration.* Cambridge, MA: Harvard University Press.

_____ (1997), *Influence and Autonomy in Psychoanalysis.* Hillsdale, NJ: The Analytic Press.

_____ (1998), Emergence of features of the analyst's life. *Psychoanal. Dial.* 8:187–194.

Mitrani, J.L. (1998), Unbearable ecstasy, reverence and awe, and the perpetuation of an "aesthetic conflict." *Psychoanal. Quart.* 67:102–127.

Pizer, S. (1992), The negotiation of paradox in the analytic process. *Psychoanal. Dial.* 2:215–240.

Price, M. (1997), The power of enactments and the enactment of power. Presented at the Fall 1997 meeting of the American Psychoanalytic Association, New York City.

Racker, H. (1968), *Transference and Countertransference.* New York: International Universities Press.

Renik, 0. (1993a), Analytic interaction: Conceptualizing technique in light of the analyst's irreducible subjectivity. *Psychoanal. Quart.* 62:553–571.

_____ (1993b), Countertransference enactment and the psychoanalytic process. In: *Psychic Structure and Psychic Change,* ed. M. Horowitz, O. Kernberg, E. Weinshel, Madison, CT: International Universities Press, pp.135–158.

_____ (1995), The ideal of the anonymous analyst and the problem of self-disclosure. *Psychoanal. Quart.* 64:466–495.

_____ (1996), The perils of neutrality. *Psychoanal. Quart.* 65:495–517.

_____ (1997), Reactions to "Observing–participation, mutual enactment, and the new classical models" by I. Hirsch. *Contemp. Psychoanal.* 33:279–284.

_____ (1998), Getting real in analysis. *Psychoanal. Quart.* 67:566–593.

Ringstrom, P.A. (1998), Therapeutic impasses in contemporary psychoanalytic treatment: Revisiting the double bind hypothesis. *Psychoanal. Dial.* 8:297–315.

Slavin, J. & Pollack, L. (1998), The struggle for recognition: Disruption and reintegration in the experience of agency. *Psychoanal. Dial.* 8: 857–873.

Slavin, M.O. & Kriegman, D., (1998) Why the analyst needs to change: Toward a theory of conflict, negotiation, and mutual influence in the therapeutic process. *Psychoanal. Dial.* 8:247–284.

Spezzano, C. (1993), *Affect in Psychoanalysis: A clinical synsthesis.* Hillsdale, NJ: The Analytic Press.

Stein, R. (1997), Review essay, "Analysis as a mutual endeavor: What does it look like?" *Psychoanal. Dial.* 7:869–880.

Stern, Donnel (1983), Unformulated experience. *Contemp. Psychoanal.* 19:71–99.

_____ (1990), Courting surprise. *Contemp. Psychoanal.* 26:452–478.

Stolorow, R., Atwood, G.E., & Ross, J. (1978), The representational world in psychoanalytic therapy. *Internat. Rev. Psycho-Anal.* 5:247–256.

Winnicott, D.W. (1969a), The use of an object and relating through identifications. In: *Playing and Reality.* New York: Routledge, 1971, pp. 86–94.

_____ (1969b), Contemporary concepts of adolescent development and their implications for higher education. *Playing and Reality.* New York: Routledge, 1971, pp. 138–150.

Wolstein, B. (1959), *Countertransference.* New York: Grune & Stratton.

32 Hawthorn Street
Cambridge, MA 02138
HollyLev@Verizon.net

"Ev'ry Time We Say Goodbye, I Die a Little … ": Commentary on Holly Levenkron's "Love (and Hate) With the Proper Stranger"

PHILIP M. BROMBERG, PH.D.

In agreement with Levenkron, I offer a postclassical psychoanalytic view of the analyst's self-revelation as part of a process that leads to the coconstruction of an intersubjective reality that incorporates the experience of each partner. When patient and analyst can each access and openly share the dissociated thoughts and feelings that are "too dangerous" to their relationship to be thought then the externalization of the patient's relationship with his own internal objects becomes available to intersubjective negotiation, self-reflection, and conflict resolution. How much self-revelation is "enough" and how much is "too much" can't be known in advance, and it is the ongoing and often painful effort to struggle with its unpredictability that defines what Levenkron calls "affective honesty," not the analyst's subjective assessment of the "truthfulness" of the personal experience she or he is considering revealing.

> Ev'ry time we say goodbye,
> I die a little;
> Ev'ry time we say goodbye,
> I wonder why, a little.
> [Cole Porter, "Ev'ry Time We Say Goodbye"]

Philip M. Bromberg, Ph.D. is a Training and Supervising Analyst, William Alanson White Institute, New York City, and Clinical Professor of Psychology, New York University Postdoctoral Program in Psychotherapy and Psychoanalysis.

I'VE OFTEN TOLD MYSELF THAT THE ONE WAY I WOULD NEVER BEGIN A commentary is "The only problem I have with this article is that I didn't write it myself." Oh, well, another broken promise. My solace is that I'm not sure I would ever have had the courage to write it. In publishing an article such as Levenkron's, an author takes a considerable risk, and I'm not referring to the risk of attacks by those who believe that there is a "correct" analytic stance and that this is not it or those who define "wild analysis" as allowing what is in your mind to come out before you have worked on it and "cleaned" it up. Even among analysts who work from a highly conservative stance, this type of allegation has few sponsors today. No, I am speaking of a different kind of risk. Since I know Holly Levenkron pretty well both personally and professionally, I know that this case presentation is not offered as a model of a routine psychoanalytic treatment, either her own or what she believes other analysts' work should look like. She chose a case that elucidates extremely vividly the power of what she terms "affective honesty"—something that she believes (as do I) is an essential part of every treatment—and in electing to present her work with her patient, Ali, she accomplishes that purpose masterfully. Because of the volatility in the transference/countertransference enactment, using this case etches her point into high relief, but it also runs the risk that analysts with leanings toward other schools of thought could read Levenkron's paper as implying that the clinical material is presented as paradigmatic—in effect saying that if affective honesty is to be respected, then relational psychoanalysis is inevitably a process of "living-through" and "working-through" volcanic enactments. This whole issue, however, fades into the background once one reflects on Levenkron's statement that "the analyst's ability to do this with someone has to be earned." Here she puts to rest the potential charge that such an analytic stance is basically an "intrusion" of the analyst's subjectivity into the patient's psychic processes and interferes with why the patient is in analysis in the first place.

At this point in the history of psychoanalysis, how Levenkron's article is read depends in part on whether a given analyst accepts that the movement from classical to postclassical theory is based on decades of clinical observation and research rather than a parochial need to supplant Freud.[1] Postclassical psychoanalysis, as clinical theory, challenges Freud's (1923)

---

[1]For a more comprehensive discussion of the classical to postclassical paradigm shift and its clinical implications, the interested reader is referred to an earlier article, "Speak to Me as to Thy Thinkings" (Bromberg, 2002).

view that human mental functioning reflects the operation of a self-contained psyche. What is being challenged is the notion that, under optimal clinical conditions, the patient's productions are generated endogenously while the analyst works with the implied (but one-sided) interaction between the patient's psyche and the analyst's presence as a fantasy object of projected imagery. This latter conceptualization of the mind has led to a set of principles as to how the analyst should conduct himself, which, in turn, has been codified as "classical technique." One central principle has been that the subjective workings of the analyst's mind should remain private and, as far as possible, be used only to organize what is ultimately offered to the patient as an interpretation. There are two reasons for this injunction against the analyst's revelation of his or her subjective mental processes: (1) because such revelation is held to be an *interference* with the analytic process, and (2) because it is held to be *unnecessary* to the analytic process. Historically, the second reason has been a relatively minor theme in classical Freudian writing because its logic has always been implied in the first reason.

In postclassical analytic theory, research, and practice, this injunction and the principle on which it is based are in the process of reevaluation. The question being most seriously discussed (as exemplified by Levenkron's case study) is not whether the analyst's "self-revelation" is "legitimate" but that it may be, a *necessary* part of the optimal analytic relationship and intrinsic to facilitating the deepest and most far-reaching growth in every patient.

Postclassical theory is moving increasingly in the direction of a psychoanalytic model of mental functioning in which our understanding of "conscious" and "unconscious" is informed by a conception of the mind as a nonlinear, relational process of meaning construction, organized by the equilibrium between stability and growth of one's self-representation; that is, by the balance between the need to preserve self-meaning (the ongoing experience of safely "being oneself") and the need to construct new meaning in the service of relational adaptation. In this model, the analyst's presence as a real person is not intentionally diminished because the concept of "endogenous unfolding" of transference projections has no valid meaning. Unconscious meaning is held to be dyadically constructed rather than "revealed." The analyst's role is not to avoid participation but to continually monitor and utilize the immediate and residual effects of participation as an inherent part of his stance.

It is from this vantage point that Levenkron's position on self-revelation must be understood: Self-revelation is the *opposite* of intrusiveness if the frame of reference of the analyst isn't that of trying to change the patient but that of sharing her own experience in order to facilitate the goal of intersubjective *negotiation* of meaning. Here, the presence of the analyst's subjective experience leading to open engagement (or confrontation) between subjectivities isn't equivalent to the classical meaning of "intrusiveness." The latter concept is derived from Freud's model of a self-contained mind that will be derailed from its optimal mode of analytic functioning by the analyst's input as a "real" person. From a postclassical perspective, open engagement between subjectivities (including open confrontation) is a necessary part of the relational context that leads to intersubjective negotiation.

Levenkron is arguing that revelation and confrontation are part of an ongoing *process* that leads to the coconstruction of a transitional reality that has room for the experience of each partner and space for negotiation. She describes this as becoming possible "when the analyst can state her point of view by offering her experience of the patient." I would add that an analyst must also try to offer, when possible, her "experience of her experience"— which frequently is a key factor that makes such revelation palatable to the patient. When the analyst reveals the elements of her internal struggle that went into deciding what to say, it reveals even more clearly that the motive for the disclosure is more one of sharing than covert indoctrination designed to *look* like sharing. I'm suggesting, in other words, that the value of affective honesty is enhanced by the analyst's openness to sharing the full complexity of her subjectivity, including her self-doubt about whether to share it. But not every confrontation can or need take that form. Let me repeat Levenkron's statement that the analyst's right to take such a stance with a patient has to be *earned*. To an analyst holding a relational view of mental growth, it is in struggling with her own limitations and self-doubts that the right to reveal her subjectivity is earned; it is in struggling with the humbling fact that she can't on her own find the "right" response; it is in struggling with her patient's experience of her while not foreclosing her own view; it is in all of this that an analyst's ability to survive intense affective confrontations and make use of them as enactments is earned, and why I believe that "earning the right to this analytic stance" is what her paper is all about.

Levenkron has written an article that I predict most analysts, regardless of theoretical creed, will appreciate, albeit, at times, nervously. She wishes to illustrate the value of "affective honesty" and "relational negotiation" as foundational analytic concepts, and in her discussion of these ideas I find the sophistication and clarity of her thinking to be inspiring. But the main reason that her argument cannot be ignored lies in the clinical material itself. The graphically detailed manner in which her interactions with her patient are presented and her generously open description of her own affectively shifting self states are such gifts to the mind and sensibility of a reader that they summon a seriously considered response. In this regard, Levenkron's writing style itself exemplifies her concept that disclosure of our thinking becomes collaborative and therefore negotiable when it is not power based.

Dissociation, Conflict, and Enactment

Enactment is not a phenomenon that speaks to a denial or an avoidance of internal conflict, but is part of the natural functioning of a mind that is simply doing what evolution has adapted it to do in terms of two discrete modes of information processing. The first, the "subsymbolic" (Bucci, 1997a, b, 2001, 2002), is organized at the level of body experience as "emotion schemas" relationally communicated through enactment; the second, the "symbolic," is organized at the level of language and conflict. When emotional experience is traumatic (more than the mind can bear), it remains unprocessed cognitively, and an automatic self-protective process takes place that results in the development of a pathological mental structure. For some people it is "a cure that is worse than the disease."

As a "fail-safe" measure to protect its own stability, the mind recruits the normal mental function of dissociation as a means of controlling the "triggering" of unprocessed emotion schemas that were created by trauma and the release of ungovernable affective hyperarousal that could threaten to destabilize its functioning. It is through the therapeutic process of helping to symbolize enacted dissociated experience that internal conflict and its potential resolution become possible. Levenkron writes, "I argue that the working through of ... enactments is not accomplished afterwards by a post hoc analysis but from within the aliveness of the experience, as part of what the patient and analyst live through together ... The problem ..." here "is that 'enacted' experiences are separated from other forms of mental process, making their analysis a separate order of thinking removed from the aliveness of the experience."

In this light, consider Bucci's (2002, p. 787) conclusions based on her research findings that "the activation of dissociated, painful experience in the session itself is central to the therapeutic process—a very different perspective from the metapsychological principle that structure depends on the inhibition of drive or desire." Bucci (2002) writes:

> The juxtaposition of subsymbolic and symbolic systems in working memory ... is central to both consciousness and the sense of self. The roots of pathology lie in dissociation within emotion schemas; *this applies at different levels to all forms of neurosis. The goal of psychoanalytic treatment is integration of dissociated schemas;* this requires activation of subsymbolic, including bodily experience, in the session itself, in relation to symbolic representations of present and past experience [p. 766, emphasis added].

This postclassical understanding of mental functioning and therapeutic growth is highly relevant to Levenkron's observation that "'revealing' ... is often a relief to the patient, even if it opens up rage and painful feelings, because it makes" clear that " ... 'being real' and connecting with another person cannot always occur through loving gestures." I believe this to be not only accurate, but a significant aspect of the relational process through which cognitive mastery of hyperaroused affective experience becomes increasingly regulated by the mind's self-reflective function. Self-regulation of dissociated, and thus potentially ungovernable, affective experience is facilitated through permitting what Bucci calls the integration of dissociated schemas that takes place through activation of subsymbolic experience in the session itself. This allows for cognitive symbolization of experience that could formerly be only enacted, and in so doing it is relieving because it increases a patient's trust in her own capacity to "think about" an otherwise overwhelming experience without the experience possessing her. Why *wouldn't* the analyst's self-revelation be relieving if it leads to increased self-reflectiveness?

In Levenkron's words, "The clinical craft ... lies in contacting a part of ourselves through which we can eventually own and reflect on either nonverbally or aloud to our patients what we have discovered about our own participation from within these interactions." This is a dimension of negotiation that "makes disclosure as 'negotiable' as any other aspect of our communications." I would put it that the relationship between what is enacted nonverbally and what is put into words during the processing of an enactment, including the analyst's revelation of her or his own subjective experience, touches on what Leston Havens (personal communication) has referred to as "Bromberg's Common Property Principle." This refers to my core belief *that the analyst's feelings about his patient are not his personal property* because they are part of a gestalt, part of an unsymbolized context within which the analyst and patient each hold pieces that are linked subsymbolically but not yet by language. During the analytic process, a main part of the analyst's job is to find words to get her own experience of this enacted communication out on the table in a manner that facilitates the patient's ability to do the same. If used judiciously, and as a negotiable element in the ongoing relationship, what has been labeled the analyst's "self-revelation" is not simply permissible and "legitimate," but a necessary part of the developmental process that Fonagy and Target (1996) call "mentalization," through which subsymbolic experience is allowed (self-reflectively) to become a part of the relational self rather than interminably enacted. There is no codified "technique" as to how this is to be accomplished with regard to the content of the mind because if one sees the mind as a nonlinear, self-organizing system, facilitation of mutative change is inherent to the *process*, not the content—a clinical observation that is consistent with the research conclusion of Lyons-Ruth and the Boston Process of Change Study Group (2001) that it is the *process* of communication ("implicit relational knowing") rather than the *content* of the communication that is the foundation for the therapeutic action of psychoanalysis. Contrary to the long held axiom of classical theory about making the unconscious conscious as a necessary condition for change, the Boston group holds that their findings support the view that *"process leads content, so that no particular content needs to be pursued; rather the enlarging of the domain and fluency of the dialogue is primary and will lead to increasingly integrated and complex content"* (Lyons-Ruth and Boston Process of Change Study Group, 2001, p. 16, emphasis added). If patient and analyst can each access and openly share the dissociated thoughts and feelings that are "too dangerous" to their relationship to be thought, then this begins to "enlarge the domain and fluency of the dialogue" and leads to "increasingly integrated and complex content" that becomes symbolized as an affective/cognitive unit and thus available to self-reflection and conflict resolution. How much self-revelation is "enough" and how much is "too much" can't be known in advance, and it is the ongoing and often painful effort to struggle with its unpredictability that defines affective honesty, not simply the analyst's subjective assessment of the "truthfulness" of the personal experience he or she is considering revealing.

Personality Development, Nonrecognition, and Shame

Having already confessed to my envy of Levenkron's courage, and having broken my resolution never to begin a commentary with my regret that I didn't write the article myself, I'm now about to risk my own neck in a manner that may turn out to be more foolhardy than courageous. Based on the early developmental history of patients like Ali with whom I myself have worked, I'm going to discuss the psychodynamics of maternal nonrecognition in creating serious dissociative mental structure in adults. In so doing, I'm going to create a story about the early personal history of *someone else's* patient—a tale of Ali and her mother that rests on intuition and "circumstantial" evidence.

Levenkron notes, "The relational or 'mutual' failings—wherein we both had to be deprived—took the form of Ali's failing to get anything from me because of her distancing and assuming behavior and my failing to take pleasure too, the pleasure commonly derived from liking another; my defenses (albeit protective) prevented me from reaching out to her in a loving way. Unless one of us shifted we would have to remain here for a while." With many patients like Ali, a key developmental issue is often the early failure of responsiveness by the mother to some genuine aspect of the child's self. This is not, necessarily, expressed through open disapproval—a response that even when cruel, communicates to the child that "who she is" at that moment has been perceptually recognized, and that what she is "doing" is being met with displeasure—but is expressed frequently through a masked withdrawal from authentic contact. This leaves the child experiencing a part of who she *is* as having no relational existence to a loved other and thus without potential pleasurable value to that other. The parent, when she dissociated from a part of the child's self—as distinguished from a manifest, fully conscious response to "bad behavior"—is implicitly communicating to the child's self that is present at that moment that she is unrecognizable as *her child*. If this type of interaction is repetitive it constitutes "cumulative developmental trauma" and leads to the creation of a dissociative mental structure that organizes the child's way of relating to herself and to the world. If it embraces too broad a segment of the core self that is formed as part of the early attachment process through mutual regulation and "implicit relational knowing" (Boston Process of Change Study Group et al., 1998), it can be the birth of annihilation anxiety.

Levenkron's account of Ali's relationship with her mother is notably brief and unelaborated, especially when compared with the lengthier and more descriptive account of the role played by Ali's father. The latter, presented in lively detail, is a picture of how Ali was a "misfit" in her family and how she tried to become a "son" to her father in response to being overshadowed by her more attractive sisters, but remained largely "unrecognized and rejected." About mother and daughter, however, Levenkron writes simply that Ali "found solace in her relationship with her mother who, *seeming to recognize Ali's style of misfitting*, co-opted her daughter into a tight, merged agreement to mutually provide love, safety, and companionship for each other." At first glance, this portrait of mutual love and closeness might appear to fit poorly with the notion of a mother's masked withdrawal from authentic contact, leaving the child experiencing herself as having no pleasurable value to a loved other. My hunch, however, is that it tends to support the above hypothesis in a way not dissimilar to the way Levenkron's difficulty in supplying details supports it. It is almost as if Ali and her mother did not have a "representable" relationship as much as a conceptualizable one, and quite the opposite is true of her relationship with her father, argumentative, confrontational, and ultimately unsatisfying though it was. The "misfit" between Ali and her father took place as a living interaction between separate people—a part of the real world that was representable mentally and verbally; but because "mis-fit" meant "misfit," for Ali to have *any* relationship with her mother they both had to assure that the "fit" was always perfect, and there is no way to do that except to foreclose separateness—what Levenkron calls "a merged agreement to mutually provide love, safety, and companionship for each other." Ali's mother, she writes, seemed "to recognize Ali's style of misfitting," and I strongly suspect this had to be true. I also suspect that the shame generated by her mother's own self-experience as a "misfit" made it impossible for her to accept her normal limitations in being able to provide what Ali needed, leading her to dissociate from the immediacy of the relationship and from the shared pleasure that it potentially held.

A powerful developmental casualty takes place when a mother dissociates her anxiety and shame to such a degree that it shuts down her ability to take pleasure in being with her child. It embodies an act of nonrecognition that is as traumatizing as the pain caused by a mother who is actively abusive, and sometimes it is *more* debilitating. Donald Fridley, a contemporary traumatologist, explicitly acknowledges (2001, p. 5) that "in many ways it is the blunt denial, disavowal, or dismissal of the child's emotional states which contributes to the child's confusion, shame, and feelings of worthlessness that has as much or more impact on the future than the fact of the physicality of the trauma itself." If the "other" systematically "*dis*confirms" (Laing, 1962) a child's state of mind, particularly at moments of intense affective arousal, by behaving as though the self-meaning of the experience to the child is either irrelevant or is "something else," the child grows to mistrust the reality of her own experience. She is impaired in her ability to cognitively process her own emotionally charged mental states in an interpersonal context—to reflect on them, hold them as states of intrapsychic conflict, and thus own them as "me." Dissociation, the disconnection of the mind from the psyche-soma, then becomes the most adaptive solution to preserving selfhood. The child's own need for *loving* recognition becomes despised and shame-ridden, a dissociated "not-me" aspect of self that, when triggered, releases not only the unmet hunger for responsiveness but a flooding of shame—the affect associated with failure of who one is, not failure in what one *does*. Failure in what one does leads to anxiety—a lowering of self-esteem, or sometimes to guilt—but it is shame that is the signal of destabilization of the *self*—the immediate or impending shock of no longer being "me." So, Ali, one might say, keeps her father's "son" always on call, ready to take over as the "tough kid" self who will protect her from the dreaded experience of revealing what she most needs to have known—that "Ev'ry time we say goodbye, I die a little ... Ev'ry time we say goodbye, I wonder why a little."

Dissociation as an Interpersonal Process

To speak to this point I need to get into the clinical material itself, and I want to focus on what to me is the most gripping, albeit complex, episode in their work together—a phase of treatment initiated by an enactment that ambushes Levenkron at a time that she is feeling particularly vulnerable. To grasp its significance to the concept of "affective honesty," it helps to recognize that even in an interaction as intensely personal as this, Levenkron has not abandoned her analytic role. Affective honesty is achieved through the analyst's *struggle* to communicate, not by a self-granted license to "tell it like it is." What comes through so clearly is that Levenkron does not grant herself such a license. Her analytic stance is organized by her comprehension that her own subjective experience does not tell her what is really going on as though it had some objective truth value. She sees its worth to the process not just in *communicating* it, but in the negotiation around whether its disclosure is experienced by her patient as an attempt to control or as an offer to share. Levenkron's dedication to balancing affective honesty with affective safety contributes powerfully to her patient's analytic growth because her attunement to her patient's safety is experienced from *within* the relationship, rather than by trying to empathically provide it as a technical stance.

The events that took place during this time are particularly compelling to me because they were so clearly framed by a major dissociative switch in self state that took place in Ali and, as so frequently happens during enactments, led to a dissociative reaction in her therapist. The self state "switching" followed Levenkron's telling Ali, unexpectedly, that she was going to take a week-long break and apologizing for the short notice. The reason for this break, unknown to Ali, was that Levenkron wished to give herself space to deal with her feelings surrounding the impending end of her seventeen-year marriage. Ali however, seeming to miss all the nonverbal cues that her therapist was in a distressed state, behaved as if she were being *gratuitously* abandoned. Levenkron put it that Ali "got in touch with the aspect of herself that, when insecure and envious, becomes filled with rage," but I feel this doesn't give quite enough weight to the magnitude of Ali's dissociative switch. To me, what happened has a different feel than someone's becoming filled with rage, which better captures the experience of a *mood* change. This seems much more of a switch in self state—fundamentally a dissociative phenomenon and not simply a change in affect—and this is what I believe made it so especially upsetting to her therapist. An affective change in itself is rarely this destabilizing to the other person; to have that kind of impact requires a switch in the entire self state that goes along with the affect. Levenkron observes Ali at that moment "turning her face to the wall and saying a few sentences that were tangential, she spoke in a slow, halted, breathy voice." This is the kind of description analysts give when they are trying to depict the nuances of what it is like to be with someone who is no longer feeling like the same person. Levenkron says that her own reaction was that of getting angry, but that she "wasn't aware of it." Why wasn't she aware of it?

As an enactment begins, an analyst will inevitably shift her self state when the patient shifts his. Dissociation is a hypnoid process, and inasmuch as analyst and patient are sharing an event that belongs equally to both of them—the interpersonal field that shapes the immediate reality of each, and the way each is experiencing herself and the other—any unsignalled withdrawal from that field by *either* person will disrupt the other's state of mind. Thus, when an enactment begins (no matter who initiates it), no analyst can be immediately attuned to the shift in here-and-now reality, and he inevitably becomes part of the dissociative process, at least for a period of time. The analyst's dissociation is not a "mistake" on his part; it is intrinsic to the normal process of human communication [Bromberg, 1996, p. 285].

Levenkron states that she began to get angrier and angrier and did not want to sooth Ali: "At that moment," she recalls, "I wanted it out on the table where I could see it." Levenkron confronts Ali angrily and Ali says "I can't stand the way you talk to me! You are so fucking mean! Who do you think you are, Holly? No one talks to me that way, only you! You're sorry for the short notice. Well what about me?" As Levenkron then puts it, "It was out on the table."

Am I saying here that I think Levenkron should have done something different? Do I think that Levenkron should have soothed her? Do I think she should have taken a different stance? No I don't. I think that the analyst entered a dissociated state of her own that was reciprocal to her patient's, and that in doing so, something unpredictable happened that ultimately became quite therapeutic. But at that moment they were in a dissociative cocoon together, so they couldn't access anything other than the dominant affect that organized their respective self states. I think Levenkron is quite explicit about that fact and states it was "as if we were a couple who was having a fight." I would argue that it wasn't "as if" they were a couple having a fight but that in their dissociative cocoon they *became* a couple having a fight.

What is most important, however, is that they weren't "just" having a fight; they were participating in an enactment that had a powerful therapeutic function because it opened space through which an analyst can come to "know" her patient and vice versa—a personal channel that is almost always very painful in this type of confrontation. Levenkron, in the heat of the "unfair" attack by Ali, found tears welling up in her eyes because she was feeling tortured by being accused of abandoning her patient to have a good time and was unable to reveal that it was just the opposite—she was taking time off to try to heal her wounds. She felt an intense need to be understood, but wasn't allowed the solace. *At that moment she was as close as she had ever been to feeling the pain of Ali's separateness and potentially self-annihilating "aloneness."* Levenkron writes that she had "a powerful urge to tell her every bad thing that ever happened to me; that is, I wanted to tell her just how hard my life had really been and how hard it certainly was at this time." The urge is poignant and Levenkron struggled with it, choosing not to act on it. Her generosity in writing about what went into the struggle takes out of the shadows what any analyst will frequently face at such a moment unless the problem is handled by a prescriptive rule—a rule that provides either a license to reveal or a prohibition against it, either of which allows the analyst to thereby sidestep this painful experience of struggle, ambivalence, and conflict.

Unlike Ali, Levenkron could not escape the pain because her own dissociative state was one in which she was "containing" some of Ali's pain. With some patients the analyst's needed participation comes about only through forcing the analyst to experience dissociated aspects of her own selfhood that lead to the recognition of dissociated aspects of the patient's self; and as this oscillating cycle of projection and introjection is processed and sorted out between them, the patient reclaims what is her own. But at that moment pain and confusion reigned for the analyst because, unlike Ali, Levenkron was forced to process simultaneously two experiences of their relationship and two self states of her own that were incompatible and irresolvable by conflict resolution. The combination of experiences was too affectively intense to be either internally or externally negotiable. "I thought I was protecting her from feeling guilty for attacking. I was also avoiding what I imagined to be a sadistic retort from her.... At that time I could not formulate what was a pull I fought against to tell all, as when the emotional and articulated demands of your patient to intrude into your privacy are so great that you 'have' to tell—for the wrong reasons." Sometimes, containing a patient's annihilating experience of saying goodbye takes an analyst to the brink of knowing what it is like to "die a little" and perhaps "wonder why, a little."

The Analyst's Right to Privacy

"Although nondisclosure here was a clear expression of my subjectivity," Levenkron comments, "I am not advancing a 'technical mandate' of nondisclosure.... In my withdrawal and silence, I was unaware of how I was enacting my self-protection and my right to privacy. I dissociated my ability to voice my boundaries—to talk to her about why I could not talk to her." Levenkron, at that moment did not reveal herself, but she is not pleased with herself for having "used nondisclosure as a foil to avoid an abuse of my privacy and admission of my vulnerability." Such a dissociative moment is part of the natural clinical process for any analyst who knows that spontaneity and aliveness ebb and flow relationally. But in her willingness to reflect on what contributed to her dissociation and to think about its various meanings of what it meant to her personally (including a wish to avoid an abuse of her privacy and admission of her vulnerability), she is here openly stating that the implications of *not* revealing are as significant to think about as those clinical moments in which an analyst *does* reveal.

I see this as quite a service to us all. In this regard, I think it important to point out that an analyst's "dissociative moments" often, as in this case, reflect not only the analyst's self-protection but also a concurrent protection of the patient. I would argue that the emotional state that Levenkron was in when she dissociated and was thereby unable to reveal "why I could not talk to her" was too affectively intense to be therapeutically usable. If she had tried to speak from that state it would have probably elevated even further Ali's already hyperaroused affect. It would have most likely reinforced Ali's dissociated "tough kid" self as her only reliable means of controlling fear and shame that would otherwise have been unregulatable. So, one could hypothesize that Levenkron's dissociation at that moment wasn't just a protection of her own *right* to privacy. It was also an adaptive relational solution to being unable to "remove myself from the explosions going off inside of me that would give me the distance I needed to speak to her in a calm way." Such a dissociation often provides a chance for things to calm down and is only problematic if the analyst uses it as a permanent hiding place rather than a temporary sanctuary.

Privacy, most simply, is a dimension of the ongoing process of negotiation between incompatible domains of self-experience. From this vantage point, the right to privacy is part of the human condition. Privacy can be surrendered by choice but not the *right* to it, and this is as true for the analyst as for the patient. Privacy and self-revelation are parts of a unitary configuration that defines the analytic relationship, for both parties, through an inevitable dialectic that takes place intrapsychically and interpersonally. My view, as I've expressed elsewhere (Bromberg, 1997), is that except for very rare instances a patient respects the analyst's personal right to privacy with regard to the analyst's history and life experiences, and in almost any situation where this *seems* not to be true, it represents a transference/ countertransference enactment in which the analyst has been unable to recognize and reveal her own dissociated experience of the patient who then, often desperately, tries to penetrate the analyst's mind to find herself within it. Let me repeat: a patient's pressure to force the analyst to give up her right to privacy is not organized by a need to simply know the analyst but to know what the analyst knows about the patient.

When an analyst is successful in her effort to "privatize" some aspect of her own experience of the patient, she is in fact depriving the patient of her potential to safely discover her own full existence—her "wholeness." The enactment then increases in power, and as the analytic space becomes filled with energy generated by this enactment, the patient more and more *becomes* the self that has been expelled from the analyst's mind, gradually forcing her way into the analyst's perceptual consciousness (Bromberg, 1998) and finally igniting in her a personal response to that part of the patient that has until then been dissociated and existed only in the enactment.

The "Personal" and the "Really Personal"

What emerges during our participation in these interactions sometimes includes the surfacing of memories or experiences from our own pasts; childhood relationships or specific events can suddenly appear, like ghosts. Often, they are ghosts we thought had been exorcised in our own analyses but that we now realize are very much *alive* in the moment and astonishingly relevant to what is taking place with that patient. What is it about these experiences that makes them such a source of debate as to how to use them? Do they fall into an austerely separate category from "process" thoughts and feelings? Are they a domain of an analyst's subjective experience that is so potentially dangerous that they should be, ipso facto, exiled from revelation, even for an analyst who might comfortably share his subjective process experience? Or, if not, how does one choose whether or not to reveal personal biographical information at such a moment? Obviously, it is a choice more complex than revelation of process feelings and seems to call forth greater concern about the welfare of not only the patient and the treatment but also about the analyst's own personal privacy.

In my view, if an analyst does disclose such information, it should be in response to a rather strong sense that it will significantly deepen the work *already* going on. I myself tend to do it only when it is part of an ongoing context in which here-and-now process experience is already being shared, and I feel strongly that it should not be done to try to *create* affective aliveness. This may be a prime clinical issue that addresses the difference between linear and nonlinear thinking in psychoanalytic theory. Like any other choice an analyst makes with a given patient, self-revelation derives its meaning from the ongoing context of the relationship in which it takes place, not from its utility as a "technique." Its usefulness to the analytic process is organized by the quality of its openness to negotiation, particularly the degree to which the analyst is free of internal pressure (conscious or unconscious) to prove his honesty or trustworthiness as a technical maneuver designed to counter the patient's mistrust. The value of an analyst's revelation of personal history rests on (1) whether what is revealed is spontaneously surfacing in the analyst's mind as part of the moment—whether it is something from her personal past that enters unbidden and very much alive into the present; (2) whether it is something that the analyst recognizes emotionally (often cognitively as well) that she was enacting while in a dissociative state of her own, and was probably a central aspect of *her* contribution to why it was so difficult to experience and respond self-reflectively to the enacted self state of her patient.

When revealing personal history I believe it is the analyst's obligation to be attuned even more sensitively than when revealing her process experience. She has to try to be aware of the even greater complexity of the patient's response to her possible motivation for the revelation, not simply to the content of what was revealed. Is the patient dissociating her own response to the analyst's behavior to keep from feeling affectively overwhelmed by what is taking place between them? This latter is a key point because an analyst's self-revelation frequently will increase a patient's dissociation, which is not an analytic error unless both analyst and patient, for too long a period of time, fail to learn something from such moments. Obviously, this bears directly on how one understands the clinical wisdom of the "strike while the iron is cold" admonition. If psychoanalytic growth is indeed a nonlinear process, it is only through *failing* to know when the temperature is right that the analyst learns when the iron is too hot and through this dialectic that the patient comes to know that the analyst is learning from her and, most importantly, cares. Simply put, by recognizing the nonlinearity of what we call "mutative change," we also accept that it does not take place through "if I do *this* correctly, then *that* will happen" but through an ineffable coming together of two minds in an unpredictable way.

Transition from Dissociation to Capacity for Conflict

As the analyst is forced to experience and respond to those aspects of the patient that both analyst and patient wished to disavow, the patient begins to inhabit a self that feels whole in the analyst's mind and thus starts to feel more simultaneously whole in her own. At that point a comfortable dialectic between subjective "insideness" and human relatedness begins to replace, for both people, the issue of right to privacy. I've called this phase of the work the transition from dissociation to capacity for conflict (Bromberg, 2001) and would like to describe it here in some detail because it is centrally important to the evolution of Levenkron's work with Ali.

In a treatment that is growth facilitating, there is increased ability to surrender the safety afforded by dissociation and a simultaneous increase in the capacity to bear and process internal conflict. A patient becomes more able, mentally, to both play with and creatively struggle with experience that before could be enacted only in the interpersonal field. In terms of clinical process, she becomes more able to "speak herself to you" as an intrapsychic process of cognitive self-symbolization that utilizes the analyst's presence as a trustworthy object. From the other end of the couch the analyst, too, starts to feel something subtly different taking place that encompasses both her experience of her patient and of herself. The analyst remains as fully engaged with her patient's immediate self state as she was when full engagement included vivid here-and-now interaction between their respective subjectivities—but now in a quieter way. If the analyst is more or less comfortably able to move with this newly developing capacity in her patient, the difference during the shift is not that collisions of subjectivity will cease but that when they do occur, the patient's self-experience is less subject to disorganization by the return of unprocessed affect. As a consequence, the patient's personality is less rigidly organized by the single dissociated truth that relational ruptures can never be repaired, and because of this the secure continuity of the attachment bond on which selfhood depends begins to be trusted as more reliable.

Levenkron's "Session 3" is an example that I think highlights the shift that takes place in the analytic work when an intersubjective space has been created by patient and therapist that permits the open processing of the collision between their individual subjectivities. Ali talks about her bodily experiences in a way that demonstrates what I've just referred to as a patient becoming more able to "speak himself to you" as an intrapsychic process of cognitive self-resymbolization that utilizes the analyst's presence as a trustworthy object. In this session, Levenkron is exquisitely attuned to Ali's affective state without needing to protect her own and is able to communicate to Ali from within this cocreated space her own thoughts about *Ali's* experience without her "otherness" being felt as a destabilizing intrusion. She is able to stay in this space with Ali, experientially, and at the same time reflect on it. "No one ever talked to you about being separate, but what is more important for us is that no one ever separated from you in a loving way."

"At this point in the session," Levenkron observes, "I was able to tell her that I hadn't realized how frightening it had been for her, but this time as she left for vacation I did feel it and said I was sorry for not understanding how scared she was of losing me. We had not talked about this openly before. I had the strangest remembrance at that moment. I recalled that when my own mother was dying, she would not let me cry; furthermore, she would not even consider that I needed to be protected in any way. She just denied her own death and wouldn't let me in on it. I was terrified, and when I later saw that I could survive her death, I wished I could have shared more with her."

This, to me, is a fascinating moment because it addresses the issue of the difference between self-revelation of "process experience" and self-revelation of "biographical data." It is one of those moments when the line between them is unusually permeable. Levenkron, apparently, did not share with Ali the spontaneous emergence of her remembrance of her mother's dying, but I could easily imagine that sharing this remembrance at that moment might have been quite therapeutic. It's one of the few moments in any clinical vignette I've read where I was able to feel the thinness of the line between the analyst's disclosing process experience and disclosing biographical data and why it is such a difficult judgment call about whether to reveal or not to reveal. Had Levenkron chosen to reveal that remembrance, it *might* have had a very positive effect in underscoring, without making explicit, the degree to which she was in close emotional contact with Ali's dissociated desire for emotional contact and was not put off by it. In other words, it could have been potentially quite shame reducing. But then again, maybe not!

Self-revelation is not a technical issue but a relational one. It has to do with the process of facilitating the construction of new mental representation, a process that is coconstructed by the participation of two minds that are alive to each other, each allowing the experience of the other to be known—a point vividly made by Anne Alvarez (1992) in her book *Live Company*. Whether an analyst chooses to reveal or chooses not to reveal is not a debate about whether or not it is reasonable to deliberately reveal something because the patient *already*, at some level, knows what you feel. If analysts accept the view that patients *do* already know what we are feeling about them as part of shared subsymbolic experience, then the primary clinical question is whether revealing it openly will or will not advance the symbolization process and lead to the construction of new mental representation (Bromberg, 2002). From this frame of reference, as Ginot (1997, p. 373) has argued cogently, "self-disclosure is not ... a way to promote a sense of intimacy through seemingly similar shared experiences. Rather, the emphasis here is on revealing emotional data growing from and organically related to the intersubjective matrix." The subjective reality of a patient's unsymbolized states of consciousness, especially with regard to a patient's experience of the analyst, must be felt and, in some useful way, acknowledged by the analyst. If there can be said to be an interpersonal or relational analytic "technique," it is mainly in the ability of the analyst throughout the course of each analysis to negotiate and renegotiate the meaning of what constitutes useful acknowledgement.

"Over time," Levenkron concludes, "Ali and I discussed our interactions with increasing comfort, partially because the development of candor is a natural evolution of any successful negotiation and partially because we both learned that articulating what we experienced did not lead to irreparable ruptures in attachment. In this light, disclosure of our thinking becomes collaborative and therefore negotiable, rather than power based." Levenkron is saying that increased analytic collaboration depends on two things: (1) *being candid is a natural part of negotiation;* it is not the application of a technical procedure that is implemented by "telling it like it is"; (2) *in the process of negotiated confrontation, the two partners learn that their confrontations do not lead to their breaking apart,* allowing the patient to more and more safely trust the reliability of a previously repudiated reality—that relational ruptures can be reparable (cf. Tronick and Weinberg, 1997).

Levenkron closes by writing, "I hope I have shown that the process of what we call 'working through an enactment', ideally, does not take place through post hoc analysis but rather that the working through is the analysis and occurs as we live it: this is the negotiation." To this I can only say, Amen.

REFERENCES

Alvarez, A. (1992), *Live Company.* London: Routledge.
Boston Process of Change Study Group, Stern, D. N., Sander, L., Nahum, J. P., Harrison, A. M., Lyons-Ruth, K., Morgan, A. C., Bruschweiler-Stern, N., & Tronick, E. Z. (1998),

Non-interpretive mechanisms in psychoanalytic therapy: The "something more" than interpretation, *Internat. J. Psycho-Anal.*, 79:903–921.

Bromberg, P. M. (1996), Standing in the spaces: The multiplicity of self and the psychoanalytic relationship. In: *Standing in the Spaces: Essays on Clinical Process,* Trauma and Dissociation. Hillsdale, NJ: The Analytic Press, 1998, pp. 267–290.

_____ (1997), The analyst's right to privacy. *Psychologist/Psychoanalyst,* 17:31–33.

_____ (1998), "Help! I'm going out of your mind." In: *Standing in the Spaces: Essays on Clinical Process, Trauma and Dissociation.* Hillsdale, NJ: The Analytic Press, 1998, pp. 309–328.

_____ (2001), The gorilla did it: Some thoughts on dissociation, the real, and the really real. *Psychoanal. Dial.,* 11:385–404.

_____ (2002), Speak to me as to thy thinkings: Some reflections on "Interpersonal Psychoanalysis' Radical Facade" by Irwin Hirsch. *J. Amer. Acad. Psychoanal.,* 30:605–620.

Bucci, W. (1997a), *Psychoanalysis and cognitive science: A multiple code theory.* New York: Guilford.

_____ (1997b), Patterns of discourse in "good" and troubled hours: A multiple code interpretation. *J. Amer. Psychoanal. Assn.,* 45:155–187.

_____ (2001), Pathways of emotional communication. *Psychoanal. Inq.,* 21:40–70.

_____ (2002), The referential process, consciousness, and sense of self. *Psychoanal. Inq.,* 22:766–793.

Fonagy, P. & Target, M. (1996), Playing with reality: I. Theory of mind and the normal development of psychic reality. *Internat. J. Psycho-Anal.,* 77:217–233.

Freud, S. (1923), The ego and the id. *Standard Edition,* 19:3–66. London: Hogarth Press, 1961.

Fridley, D. (2001), Critical Issues: attachment and dissociative disorders. *Internat. Soc. for Study of Dissoc. News,* 19:4–5.

Ginot, E. (1997), The analyst's use of self, self-disclosure, and enhanced integration. *Psychoanal. Psychol.,* 14:365–381.

Laing, R. D. (1962), *The Self and Others.* Chicago: Quadrangle.

Lyons-Ruth, K. & Boston Process of Change Study Group. (2001), The emergence of new experiences: Relational improvisation, recognition process, and non-linear change in psychoanalytic therapy. *Psychologist-Psychoanalyst,* 21:13–17.

Tronick, E. Z. & Weinberg, M. K. (1997), Depressed mothers and infants: Failure to form dyadic states of consciousness. In: *Postpartum Depression and Child Development,* ed. L. Murray & P. Cooper. New York: Guilford, pp. 54–81.

300 Central Park West
New York, NY 10024

Affective Experiences and Honesty in the Interaction: Discussion of Holly Levenkron's Paper

JAMES L. FOSSHAGE, PH.D.

Anchoring her views in the work of Benjamin and other American relational authors, Levenkron asserts that intersubjective relatedness in which there is recognition of separate realities is essentially the only form of relatedness. Framing growth as coming about through the recognition of another's subjectivity provides a basis for "confrontation" and for a more direct injection of the analyst's subjectivity into the analytic encounter. More specifically, it fosters the expression of the analyst's subjectivity from what this author calls the "other-centered" and "self" perspectives.

In contrast, the recognition of selfobject and caretaking relatedness positions the analyst to express directly aspects of the analyst's subjectivity pertaining to mirroring, idealizing, and twinship selfobject needs. Kohut and classical self psychologists have delineated selfobject needs and the selfobject dimension of relatedness and transference and have emphasized the consistent use of the empathic listening/experiencing perspective. American relational theorists have delineated intersubjective relatedness and the usefulness of the other-centered listening/experiencing perspective. This author focuses on an integrative theory including three forms of relatedness and different listening/experiencing perspectives. Different listening/experiencing perspectives and forms of relatedness fundamentally influence analysts' affective experiences within the analytic encounter as exemplified in Levenkron's case.

James L. Fosshage, Ph.D. is President, International Association for Psychoanalytic Self Psychology; Co-founder and Faculty, National Institute for the Psychotherapies and Institute for the Psychoanalytic Study of Subjectivity (NYC); Clinical Professor, New York University Postdoctoral Program in Psychotherapy and Psychoanalysis.

THIS, PERHAPS MORE THAN MANY, IS A DEEPLY PERSONAL PAPER. Personal in the sense that Holly Levenkron presents, largely through her case illustration, her views on the nature of the psychoanalytic enterprise—the nature of the engagement, its tone, its character, and the crucial elements that make for change.

It has emerged more clearly than ever that to be effective an analytic relationship requires a deep emotional engagement between patient and analyst. The ongoing paradigmatic shifts from objectivism to constructivism and from intrapsychic to relational field theories have provided the conceptual footholds for this realization. Levenkron adds to the growing literature in delineating important features of an analytic interaction, focusing specifically on enactment, intersubjective relatedness, and affective honest communication. She further delineates these features in her case illustration, meaningfully amplified through her sharing detailed subjective experiences of both patient and analyst.

While relational theorists (including analysts from interpersonal, object relational, self psychological, and American relational perspectives) share a good deal in theory and technical guidelines, we also differ as much (Fosshage, 2003). Alternative perspectives provide different angles, different lenses, different understandings, and different clinical interactions. I refer to my conceptual tilt as relational self psychology or contemporary self psychology. Like most contemporary self psychologists and intersubjectivists (for example, Stolorow, Brandchaft, and Atwood, 1987; Lichtenberg, Lachmann, and Fosshage, 1992, 1996, 2002; Bacal, 1998; Shane, Shane, and Gales, 1998; Lachmann and Beebe, 2002; Stolorow, Atwood, and Orange, 2002), I conceive of the analytic relationship as an interactive system formed by patient and analyst and their respective subjectivities. I have emphasized in my own writing how the analytic relationship, involving complex implicit and explicit processing, is coconstructed and requires of both patient and analyst deep emotional engagement to illuminate and to create new relational experience (implicit relational knowledge) (Fosshage 1994, 1995b; Lichtenberg, Lachmann, and Fosshage, 2002).

Thus, I am in full agreement with Holly Levenkron's depiction of the therapeutic requisites of a powerful emotional engagement between patient and analyst, importantly including what she calls affective honest communication. I believe, however, that with her exclusive focus on intersubjective relatedness, she overlooks other forms of relatedness. Moreover, I disagree with her depiction of intersubjective relatedness as inherently adversarial.

I will first address the following conceptual issues: intersubjective relatedness: "a collision of realities"; selfobject and care-taking relatedness; the influence of listening/experiencing perspectives on an analyst's affective experience; and enactments. I will then track the clinical material and contrast Levenkron's perspective with my own.

Intersubjective Relatedness: "A Collision of Realities"

Intersubjective relatedness, as delineated by Stern (1985) and Benjamin (1988, 1990), refers to a growth-promoting recognition of the separate subjectivity of the other. Most American relational authors tend to view intersubjective relatedness as the only form of relatedness (an exception is Slochower, 1996, with her use of Winnicott's concept of holding environment). Levenkron likewise focuses exclusively on intersubjective relatedness.

Levenkron views intersubjective relatedness as inherently adversarial (an aspect emphasized by Slavin and Kriegman from an evolutionary biological perspective, 1992). She notes Benjamin's (1990) suggestion of a fundamental paradox in recognition—"a constant tension between recognizing the other and asserting the self." She then describes the patient and analyst encounter as a "collision of realities", a "colliding of [their] agendas." "Each person," according to Levenkron, "tries to change the other in terms of their own conscious and unconscious agendas. ... We inevitably push against each other's realities." To achieve "intersubjective space, each person has to surrender 'some' of the hold each has on her own subjectivity in order to pay attention to the other, even if that *other's view is opposed to her own, (and it has to be, simply because it's different)*" (my italics).

Levenkron captures an aspect of all relationships and, more specifically, all analytic relationships—that is, at one time or another all relationships, because of differences in subjectivities, are experienced as conflicting, adversarial, and oppositional. Recognition of differences in subjectivities, however, can generate other types of experiences. For example, differences can be experienced as interesting, expanding, growth producing, and self-delineating. An analyst's "belief" that relationships are inherently adversarial, as with any belief, will certainly shape the analytic or intersubjective (relatedness) encounter.

Levenkron does depict an avenue of resolving the conflicting differences:

> To whatever degree we give up our tight hold on our own subjectivity, we increase the potential to validate the other person's subjectivity, while retaining our own. As we are doing this, the experience of relatedness to the other person increases, as can the experience of learning and of loving.

In contrast, experience amply demonstrates from my vantage point that our subjectivity variably facilitates or encumbers comprehension of another's subjectivity. Moreover, each of us varies from moment to moment as to flexibility and openness to the recognition of another's subjective experience. When Levenkron refers to "our tight hold on our subjectivity," I believe that she is capturing those moments when primary attitudes (organizing patterns, implicit mental models, expectancies) are activated, and they interfere with the recognition and understanding of a patient's subjective experience. Instead of recognitive understanding, these primary attitudes and corresponding neural memory networks (Nelson, 1986; Edelman, 1987) have us in their "grips." These moments, as Levenkron describes, require us to become aware of the particular encumbering attitude to be able to relinquish "our tight hold" and to hear, recognize, and implicitly "validate" the patient's subjectivity.

In developing her motivational model, Levenkron begins with positing that to get our needs met is a basic human striving—fair enough. Yet, she limits the needs to "getting the object of our desire, more specifically, getting the object of our own desire to recognize us." Interestingly, to get the other to recognize us corresponds with mirroring selfobject needs—that is, a need for acknowledgment, recognition, and affirmation from the other (Kohut, 1971, 1984). While certainly both patient and analyst experience variable selfobject needs with regard to each other (Bacal and Thomson, 1996), and with variable intensity, to limit our needs to the recognition from the other inadvertently sets up, once again, an adversarial quality to the analytic encounter in which both participants aim "to get their individual needs met."

In contrast to Levenkron's model, Lichtenberg (1989) has made a case for at least five basic needs that emerge and develop into variably functional or dysfunctional motivational systems. In addition, I believe that within the attachment motivational arena, relational needs are more complex; they include not only needs for intersubjective relatedness but also needs for selfobject and care-taking relatedness—a topic I will now address.

Selfobject and Care-Taking Relatedness

While American relational authors have importantly delineated intersubjective relatedness as a primary form of relatedness, Kohut (1971, 1984) and self psychologists have described a second primary form of relatedness, what I (Fosshage, 1997) call "selfobject relatedness" and Shane, Shane, and Gales (1998) call "self with self-transforming other dimension." Selfobject relatedness involves the use of the other for purposes of self-regulation. Kohut identified three types of selfobject needs, called mirroring, idealizing, and twinship selfobject needs. When the patient's selfobject needs are in the forefront, the patient is interested in very specific aspects of the analyst's subjectivity.[1] For example, the patient may want to know how the analyst feels about the patient: "Do you like me?" "Do you care about me?" "Will you protect me?" "Can I feel safe with you?" "Do you have qualities that I admire and can use as ideals and incentives for my own growth?"

A third primary form of relatedness involves focusing on the concerns or needs of the other, what I call care-taking relatedness—for example, a parent's care-taking of a child, a teacher with a student, an analyst with a patient. Care-taking is based on our empathic capacity to resonate with the affects, identify the experience, and understand the needs of the other. From an evolutionary biological perspective, Ronald Lee (2003) at the University of California at Berkeley in a recent and what is considered a path-breaking paper links parenting or giving to others with aging, that is, the biological reason we live longer is to give or provide parental (and grandparental) care.

Relational needs and forms (or dimensions) of relatedness shift in priority during analytic work for each analyst as well as patient. When the pa-

[1]Based on Kohut's original formulation of archaic merger (no longer viable in light of Dan Stern's, 1985, view that self and object differentiation exists at birth), a common misunderstanding is that selfobject relatedness does not involve a separate other. Selfobject relatedness does involve a separate other but the patient is interested in very specific aspects of the analyst's subjectivity related to self-regulation (see Fosshage, 1992, 2003, for further explanation).

tient's selfobject needs are in the foreground the patient requires the analyst to be reciprocally concerned with the patient, a care-taking relatedness. These complementary needs and forms of relatedness create, not conflict ("to get their needs met") between the patient and analyst, as Levenkron suggests, but a mutually enhancing interaction. When a patient's selfobject needs and relatedness are in the foreground, a fuller expression of the analyst's subjectivity and needs (for example, the analyst's need for intersubjective relatedness or selfobject relatedness), however, can easily usurp analytic space and thwart the patient's selfobject needs, disrupting the interaction. A patient's need for intersubjective relatedness requires reciprocal intersubjective relatedness from the analyst and probably a fuller disclosure of the analyst's subjectivity. An analyst's withholding of his subjectivity can thwart the patient's needs for intersubjective relatedness, preventing a growth-promoting moment of mutual recognition. And, when a patient expresses concern for the analyst (for example, the analyst's fatigue, illness, or the loss of an important other), the analyst is required to be reciprocally comfortable with his or her selfobject needs coming to the fore and with receiving a patient's care-taking. These shifts in forms of relatedness for patient and analyst are often quite seamless in a foreground/background configuration. To include in our theory of attachment three forms of relatedness, as compared to only one (for example, only selfobject relatedness in classical self psychology and only intersubjective relatedness in American relational theory), enables the analyst to understand and relate to the patient's, as well as his or her own, shifting priority of needs (Fosshage, 1997, 2003; Shane, Shane, and Gales, 1998).

The Influence of Listening/Experiencing Perspectives on an Analyst's Affective Experience

Many factors influence analysts' subjective experiences of patients, including analysts' listening/experiencing perspectives. As our listening/experiencing perspective shifts, our subjective experience and "affective honesty" also changes. We cannot talk about affective honesty in the singular, for our affective experiences can quickly shift as we move from one listening/experiencing perspective to another.

Listening and experiencing as well as possible through affect resonance and vicarious introspection from within the frame of reference of the patient is what Kohut (1959, 1982) called the empathic perspective. That is, the empathic perspective positions an analyst to attempt to understand the patient's experience from within the patient's perspective.

For the analyst to experience a patient as "an other" in relationship with the patient—what it feels like to be the other person in that relationship—is what I have called the other-centered perspective (Fosshage, 1995a, 1997). When we describe a patient as hostile, controlling, demanding, or loving, we are experiencing the patient from the perspective of the other in a relationship with the patient. When a patient expresses intense affect, love, or anger toward the analyst, the analyst typically experiences himself as the other in a relationship with the patient from the other-centered perspective. While the empathic perspective potentially informs us about the patient's experience, the other-centered perspective potentially informs us about the patient's old or newly emergent relational (self with other) patterns.

The impact of these differing perspectives on the analyst's experience and understanding of the patient, serving as the basis for the analyst's responding, cannot be overstated. They create very different clinical moments. In my view, we need to use both perspectives to enhance our comprehension of our patients and their relationships. In addition, I have proposed that an overriding use of the empathic mode, whether in the foreground or background, helps us to assess how and when to use information from each of these perspectives therapeutically and helps to guide us in the interaction.

Whereas both the empathic and other-centered perspectives are focused on the patient, I have recently added a third perspective—what I call the analysts's self perspective (Fosshage, 2003). While analysis entails a primary focus on the analysand, what may come to the forefront for the analyst is her or his own perspective that, rather than emanating out of an empathic or other-centered patient focus, reflects the analyst's self experience. An analyst may either use his self-perspective internally or share directly his perspective in a variety of clinical situations. For example, in attempting to understand who is contributing what to a patient/analyst interaction, an analyst must independently assess, as best as he can, his subjective experience during that interaction.

When Levenkron speaks of affective honesty, to know, and to be able to choose, from what listening/experiencing perspective we are experiencing the patient can help us facilitate the analytic process. For example, we might experience a patient from an other-centered perspective as demanding and controlling, informing us about relational patterns. If we are able to shift into an empathic perspective, however, we might experience the patient in the same interaction as desperate and in need of feeling loved or cared for, important issues that need to be addressed. Both experiences are affectively honest. The art is to be able to use these different perspectives flexibly in a growth-promoting manner. While a "tight hold on our own subjectivity" might be from any one of these perspectives, I believe that we more easily get "stuck" in other-centered and self perspectives. To be able to move from one perspective to another provides an opportunity to loosen the "tight hold."

Enactments

For Levenkron, negotiating enactments is central to the analytic process. To define enactment she borrows Renik's (1997) usage, "there is only enactment (singular), a constant, unavoidable aspect of everything patient and analyst do in analysis" (p. 282). While Levenkron states that "enactment exists at all times as the substrate of analytic interaction", in using Renik's definition enactment becomes synonymous with interaction. Why does Levenkron refer to enactment as a "substrate of analytic interaction"? She seems to be emphasizing the unconscious, dissociated aspects of both parties participating in enactments, and their subsequent coming into conscious awareness, as central to her theory of analytic change.

In an interaction systems model, everything in the analytic encounter is interaction. We cannot differentiate between action ("acting-in," "acting-out") and articulation, for the latter is also action. Thus, within an interaction systems model, we differentiate between nonverbal and verbal actions and communications. Within this model, I have defined enactments as affectively poignant interactions that can be positive and/or negative, conscious and/or unconscious (Fosshage, 1995b).

Levenkron makes clear that "working-through" of enactments "is not accomplished afterwards, by a post hoc analysis, but from within the aliveness of the experience, as part of what patient and analyst live through together." In other words when we are in the throes of an enactment, especially those interactions that involve aversiveness, usually we can only find our way out through opening up the reflective process for mutual exploration. This mutual exploration requires each participant's honest disclosure of her/his respective affective experiences. I am in total agreement with Levenkron with this description and technical guideline, for I find that to emerge from disruptions that become impasses requires each participant to put their feelings and thoughts "on the table" to sort out who is contributing what to the interaction.

Ali and Holly and Their Analytic Interaction

To address another analyst's clinical material I find to be invigorating, but daunting. It is invigorating to see and attempt to understand another analyst's work and to compare it with one's own take on the matter. It is daunting, for I, as a reader was not present and did not personally experience the complex affective communicative exchanges. Because of space limitations we get a limited glimpse of the analysis. In addition, we neither hear the intonations and inflections nor see the accompanying nonverbal expressions that amplify and nuance the communicative exchange. Moreover, each analyst–patient dyad is unique; our comments from the outside make it a different analysis.

With that said, I will share some of my reactions to the complex clinical material that Holly Levenkron has provided us. She has rendered this material with considerable openness about her ongoing subjective experience as well as that of the patient's, which better enables us, even from the outside, to enter the exchange. I will track the sessions, commenting on them as presented and offering at times alternative formulations. I will also use the first names of patient and analyst, better representing the type of relational analytic encounter (using relational as a broad rubric) that Holly Levenkron is presenting. The analytic structure and patients' constructions notwithstanding, a relational analytic encounter tends to create a more level, rather than hierarchical, playing field between analyst and patient than is customary in traditional psychoanalysis.

The Lobby Encounter

Ali's "bold" comment about Holly's "great legs" that sexually aroused her triggered in Holly an uncomfortable sense of intrusion. Holly experienced Ali's comment as aggressive, entitled, and controlling. It stifled Holly's capacity to enjoy the compliment, to be playful, and even flirtatious. It also stifled for a time a fuller exploration (from an empathic perspective) of what Ali was experiencing.

Holly says, "Ali was assuming a relationship I was not offering." To me, it was not clear what kind of relationship Ali wanted. Holly said that she had to fail Ali's selfobject needs, for she did not want to meet them. Yet, it was not clear what Ali's selfobject needs were or if they were in the foreground of Ali's experience. For a moment Holly attempts to enter empathically into Ali's subjectivity: "I experienced her expressions as, "I need you to desire me—I need to have a certain significance to you that requires you to put aside your own self—your own subjectivity." Framing Ali's mirroring selfobject needs as requiring Holly to put aside her own self, however, lends itself to a feeling of being controlled from the other-centered perspective. Later, Holly returns to an empathic perspective and "came to see it was about her wish and fantasy that I desire her to desire me. This was conveyed to me in her remark, "C'mon Holly, you wanted me to look at your legs and you know it."

While an empathic perspective is an *attempt* to understand from within the patient's frame of reference, it is, of course, invariably shaped by our models and other aspects of our subjectivity that can render our understandings as more or less accurate from the patient's perspective. Rather than Ali's desiring Holly to desire her, her comment, "C'mon Holly, you wanted me to look at your legs and you know it," could have been Ali's expectancies, based on her experience with her sisters. In addition I suspect that Holly, reminding Ali of her feminine sisters, triggered Ali's competitiveness and envy and in turn the aggression Holly felt.

Holly's experience of Ali's remark as aggressive and intrusive required Holly to self-regulate and to momentarily forfeit empathic inquiry. At such moments, our ability to be able to move into empathic inquiry, though not always available, can create the pause needed for self-regulatory efforts. It can, as well, help to enlarge our view as to what just took place. Nevertheless, the information gained from the other-centered perspective provided important information about Ali's relational patterns involving attractive feminine women and relational history especially, I believe, related to her feminine sisters. The dance in the use of these two listening/experiencing perspectives provides for a more comprehensive understanding of the patient.

Viewing Ali's actions as more generally involving love and caring, Holly experienced Ali's "demands" for caring as aggressive, controlling, and stifling. From an empathic perspective, Ali's desperate need for caring probably emanates from her expectancies based on the relationship with her father that the other person, now in this case Holly, does not love her. From an other-centered perspective, Holly understandably experienced her "demands" for love as stifling, inadvertently preventing Holly's love from emerging. Using empathic and other-centered garnered information, Holly subsequently spells out how Ali's aggression, used actively in her relationship with her father, enabled her to connect to her father as well as to protect herself against vulnerability involving her desires for tenderness and her expectancies of disappointment. Holly notes Ali's expectancies of not getting love and caring, and Ali's subsequent attempts to demand or to take love and caring that stifles the other person. In an act of self-assertion, Holly affirms that she wants to give Ali love and caring, but "you just have to let me do that in my own time." Ali was moved to tears with the illumination of this struggle, with Holly's open and honest disclosure of her experience and assertion of her needs (aspects of intersubjective relatedness), and with Holly's clear expression of caring for Ali (responding to Ali's selfobject needs). Ali had found a person who, unlike her father, was cooperative, caring, and desiring to have an intimate relationship with her.

Holly and Ali were forging new relational experience that would serve as the basis for the formation of new expectancies (implicit relational knowledge, Stern et al., 1998). Holly points out that her interpretative comments emanated from within the struggle with an affective honesty that served as a "powerful source of therapeutic action." I certainly agree. I would add that her interpretive understanding, emanating from both her other-centered and empathic experience, made it more comprehensive and usable to the patient; to have remained solely in the other-centered perspective could have resulted in a communicative impasse.

The enactment, in my view, was a poignant interaction to which patient and analyst variably contributed. Exploring the incident and honestly articulating their respective experiences enabled analyst and patient to create more reflective space in which the relational scenario was understood and, simultaneously, a new relational experience was being cocreated.

Just after Ali had experienced Holly as loving, Ali became fearful of losing Holly—"Now I feel as if you're going to leave me,." The emergence of Ali's fear of Holly's abandonment, in my view, might have been connected to her mother, with whom intimacy was always tinged with her mother's anxiety and insecurity. Ali's mother apparently had often required a merger-like experience in an attempt to quell the anxiety—creating expectancies in Ali (dreaded, yet familiar and desired) of a merger-like experience in her relationship with Holly.

Holly directly reassured her and kept the relational pattern in focus: "I'm here, I'm not going anywhere. But you can push me away if you insist I give you all of me." Holly's honest reassurance was a direct response to Ali's selfobject need for a protective, caring other (unlike mother). Holly's recognition of Ali's potential participation of demanding from Holly increased, I suspect, Ali's awareness and sense of personal agency.

A Bleak Friday

In a precarious, exhausted, and vulnerable state Holly announces a week's vacation and apologizes for a short notice. She explains that "something personal had happened that had to be dealt with." Despite the tone of this, Ali is riveted to her construction (the historical basis of which is not clear, but possibly related to her experiences with father and her sisters) that wonderful things are happening to Holly. She feels unimportant to Holly and is deflated (a selfobject rupture). Then, using aggression to bolster self-assertion, Ali laments, "You're sorry for the short notice, well, what about me?" In my view, Ali felt that she didn't count, that she wasn't important to Holly. In her world, for example, her sisters received the needed affirmation and she didn't. When in the grips of this implicit mental model, other potentially contradictory cues (for example, Holly said something had happened and had to be dealt with—a seemingly ominous cue) are not attended to, and she constructs current reality in keeping with the repetitive experience of the past.

When traumatic patterns of organization are activated, a patient such as Ali can be relentless for, to the patient, the trauma is being replicated and the betrayal is powerful. Holly could not disclose her reasons for the short notice undoubtedly because they were too personal and painful. In the face of Ali's rage and implicit demands, Holly understandably experienced that self-disclosure would have been an act of subjugation and relational suicide. The bind, however, is that the absence of disclosure feeds the patient's conviction that the patient is right—the trauma is being repeated. In this instance, it was not clear from the protocol how Holly and Ali emerged from this difficult moment. Holly did become aware, retrospectively, that she had lost her ability, probably related to her personal stress, "to talk to her about why I could not talk to her," again the very avenue that helped them emerge from the previous problematic enactment.

Session Three: "I Want to be Missed"

Just as Ali was to go on vacation, she turned to Holly and said, "I hope you'll be all right." Remembering her own surgery during one separation, Holly empathically inquired "What is it?" Ali replied, "Well, I'm worried you may get sick—your heart." Ali's expression of her fear triggered an empathic resonance in Holly. Holly directly reassures her—an empathic response (that is, a response based on her empathic understanding of what Ali needed). To my ears, two people are sensitively talking and relating to one another. Ali's fear and selfobject needs for a protective other are in the foreground (selfobject relatedness). Holly remains empathically focused and is protective (caretaker relatedness). This is a good example of when a patient's selfobject needs are in the forefront, a patient is interested in a very specific aspect of the analyst's subjectivity. To reiterate, an analyst functioning as a caretaker at these moments best complements the patient's selfobject relatedness.

Upon her return Ali grinned and said, "So! You survived my absence, Holly? You didn't die without me!" Something in her statement challenged Holly, triggering aversiveness. Holly's question, "Is your grin telling me something?", feels cautious and aversively tinged, leading to Ali's with-drawal and silence. Holly then asked, from a more empathic perspective but perhaps still slightly aversive (depending on the intonation and the de-gree to which Holly at this moment experienced Ali's desires as demand-ing), "Did you *want* to hear that I couldn't live without you?" Ali quickly takes the opening, "Yes, that's true. I wanted you to miss me, to hold me in your thoughts the way I think about you. To think about me all the time and wish I were here." She then adds, "I was upset when I left! You didn't seem to care enough." Disheartened Ali began to wonder if she were progressing in therapy. Holly noted that she felt further threatened by Ali's disparage-ment of treatment and movement toward withdrawal.

Ali stated that she very much wanted to be missed totally (like a mother with a daughter) so that she *knew* that she was important to Holly. As a leg-acy from her past, Ali remained in doubt about her importance to Holly and was striving to consolidate a sense of importance and value (what Kohut re-ferred to as the leading edge of the material, that is, what the patient is striv-ing toward; Miller, 1985; Tolpin, 2002). Depending on our self states, mod-els, and listening/experiencing perspectives, our reaction to Ali at this moment could be quite varied. Holly, with her focus on intersubjective re-latedness and the use of the other-centered perspective, experienced Ali's wish to be an unrealistic demand that constricted her and her love for Ali. In my view, Holly's experience of Ali prevented her at this juncture from playing and cocreating a "transitional space" (Winnicott, 1965), a moment of resonance between them involving Ali's desire to be missed and important to her analyst.

In addition to Ali's need to be important to Holly, the separation might also have triggered a relational (transference) pattern in which her mother needed her to quell her own anxiety and insecurity, what Ali might have experienced as oppressive but also as providing a reassuring tie (an anxious attachment). While there did not seem to be much evidence of the activation of this theme, clearly Holly's not needing her in the same way could have been experienced both as a bit anxiety producing (a threat to an attachment pattern) and as relieving (cocreating new implicit relational experience).

Ali's need to have been missed and to be important and Holly's experience of Ali as demanding and controlling created a difficult impasse. Holly opens it up for inquiry, involving exploration and, once again, honest revelation of her own subjective experience as well as the patient's. Holly depicts Ali's wish to be missed as an unrealistic demand that constricts Holly and her love for Ali.

It becomes clear that Holly and Ali have seen Ali's "need to merge" pejoratively. As indicated, I suspect Ali's need to merge is a learned attachment pattern, for anxious mothers tend to breed anxious daughters (Main, 2000). She is attempting to find safety (Bowlby, 1969) and to feel valued (Kohut, 1971). The developmental process is not separation–individuation (Mahler, Pine, and Bergman, 1975) but attachment–individuation (Lyons-Ruth, 1991). Secure attachment increases self-regulatory capacity and creates confidence in attachment and interactive regulation (Beebe and Lachmann, 2002).

Ali's concern that her "fears can never end" triggered an empathically resonating response in Holly. Framing this in terms of separation, Holly and Ali arrive at how Ali's mother never showed her "that you can be safe even if you are separate." The discussion turns to death and Ali's fear that she could never be able to bear Holly's death. Ali spoke of feeling "really basically okay, yet all she wanted to do was to be curled up in my womb." Her wish to be in Holly's womb, I believe, was her attempt to use Holly to allay her anxiety and secure a sense of safety. Holly directly asserts her reassuring belief that Ali could survive it, recognizing "that no one ever separated from you in a loving way." Holly's belief in Ali's capacity to survive provided the basis for new relational experience and new implicit relational knowledge. Aversiveness subsides, the logjam is broken, the rupture is repaired, new understanding and an empathic reassuring resonance emerge.

Conclusion

Anchoring her views in the work of Benjamin and other American relational authors, Levenkron asserts that intersubjective relatedness in which there is recognition of separate realities is essentially the only form of relatedness. Framing growth as coming about through the recognition of another's subjectivity provides a basis for "confrontation" and for a more direct injection of the analyst's subjectivity into the analytic encounter. More specifically, it fosters the expression of the analyst's subjectivity from other-centered and self perspectives.

In contrast, the recognition of selfobject and caretaking relatedness positions the analyst to directly express aspects of the analyst's subjectivity pertaining to mirroring, idealizing, and twinship selfobject needs. For example the analyst, as did Levenkron, may implicitly or explicitly affirm, reassure, be protective, and provide ideals.

Kohut and classical self psychologists have delineated selfobject needs and the selfobject dimension of relatedness and transference. They have emphasized the consistent use of the empathic listening/experiencing perspective. American relational theorists have delineated intersubjective relatedness and the usefulness of what I call the other-centered listening/experiencing perspective. Contemporary self psychologists have focused on a broader theory including varied forms of relatedness (Fosshage, 1997; Shane, Shane, and Gales, 1998) and different listening/experiencing perspectives (Lichtenberg, 1984; Fosshage, 1995a, 2003).

In my view, an analyst who functions with a singular notion of intersubjective relatedness potentially can thwart and disrupt the patient's selfobject needs. Entering from the other-centered and the analyst's self perspectives can usurp the space needed for the emergence of selfobject needs. Partially for these reasons Levenkron, in my view, had difficulty in joining the patient in her wish and need to feel missed by her analyst. Levenkron could not, of course, belie her subjectivity; yet, a more inclusive model, I believe, would have enabled her to create the needed transitional space to join the patient in the spirit that "of course Ali would want her to miss her and know that she is important to her."

That notwithstanding, I am in full agreement with Levenkron's thesis that an open and honest sharing of respective subjective experiences provides the most reliable avenue for emerging from those enactments that have become impasses. When patient and analyst are interlocked in a way that shuts down the process, the most facilitative way out is to raise the whole process—the subjective experience of each participant in the interaction—for an open and honest inquiry. In this process, analyst and patient can begin to feel heard and that, in turn, enables each to enter reflectively into the other's experience (the empathic perspective) and to arrive at an understanding of one another.

REFERENCES

Bacal, H. ed. (1998), *How Therapists Heal Their Patients: Optimal Responsiveness.* Northvale, NJ: Jason Aronson.
_____ & Thomson, P.G. (1996), The psychoanalyst's selfobject needs and the effect of their frustration on the treatment: a new view of countertransference. In: *Basic Ideas Reconsidered: Progress in Self Psychology,* Vol. 12, ed. A. Goldberg. Hillsdale, NJ: The Analytic Press, pp. 17–34.
Beebe, B. & Lachmann, F. (2002), *Infant Research and Adult Treatment.* Hillsdale, NJ: The Analytic Press.
Benjamin, J. (1988), *The Bonds of Love.* New York: Pantheon Press.
_____ (1990), An outline of intersubjectivity: The development of recognition. *Psychoanal. Psychol.,* 7:33–46.
Bowlby, J. (1969), *Attachment and Loss. Vol. 1, Attachment.* London: Hogarth Press.
Edelman, G. (1987), *Neural Darwinism: The Theory of Neural Group Selection.* New York: Harper & Row.
Fosshage, J. (1992), Self psychology: the self and its vicissitudes within a relational matrix. In: *Relational Perspectives in Psychoanalysis,* eds. N. Skolnick & S. Warshaw. Hillsdale, NJ: The Analytic Press, pp. 21–42.
_____ (1994), Toward reconceptualizing transference: theoretical and clinical considerations. *Internat. J. Psycho-Anal.,* 75:265–280.
_____ (1995a), Countertransference as the analyst's experience of the analysand: Influence of listening perspectives. *Psychoanal. Psychol.,* 12:375–391.
_____ (1995b), Interaction in psychoanalysis: A broadening horizon. *Psychoanal. Dial.,* 5:459–478.
_____ (1997), Listening experiencing/perspectives and the quest for a facilitating responsiveness. In: *Conversations in Self Psychology, Progress in Self Psychology,* Vol. 13, ed. A. Goldberg. Hillsdale, NJ: The Analytic Press, pp. 33–55.
_____ (2003), Contextualizing self psychology and relational psychoanalysis: Bi-directional influence and proposed syntheses. *Contemp. Psychoanal.,* 39:411–448.
Kohut, H. (1959), Introspection, empathy and psychoanalysis. *J. Amer. Psychoanal. Assn.,* 7:459–483.
_____ (1971), *The Analysis of the Self.* New York: International Universities Press.

_____ (1982), Introspection, empathy, and the semicircle of mental health. *Internat. J. Psycho-Anal.,* 63:395–408.

_____ (1984), How Does Analysis Cure? ed. A. Goldberg & P. Stepansky. Chicago: University of Chicago Press.

Lee, R. (2003), Why we die, why we live: A new theory of aging. Reported by Nicholas Wade, The Science Times, *The New York Times,* July 15, 2003, p. F3.

Lichtenberg, J. (1984). The empathic mode of perception and alternative vantage points for psychoanalytic work. In: *Empathy II,* eds. J. Lichtenberg, M. Bornstein, & D. Silver. Hillsdale, NJ: The Analytic Press, pp. 113–136.

_____ (1989), *Psychoanalysis and Motivation.* Hillsdale, NJ: The Analytic Press.

_____, Lachmann, F., & Fosshage, J. (1992), *Self and Motivational Systems: Toward a Theory of Technique.* Hillsdale, NJ: Analytic Press.

_____, Lachmann, F., & Fosshage, J. (1996), *The Clinical Exchange: Technique from the Standpoint of Self and Motivational Systems.* Hillsdale, NJ: The Analytic Press.

_____, Lachmann, F., & Fosshage, J. (2002), *A Spirit of Inquiry: Communication in Psychoanalysis.* Hillsdale, NJ: The Analytic Press.

Lyons-Ruth, K. (1991), Rapprochement or approchement: Mahler's theory reconsidered from the vantage point of recent research on early attachment relationships. *Psychoanal. Psychol.,* 8:1–23.

Mahler, M., Pine, F., & Bergman, A. (1975), *The Psychological Birth of the Human Infant.* New York: Basic Books.

Main, M. (2000), The organized categories of infant, child, and adult attachment: Flexible vs. inflexible attention under attachment-related stress. *Journal of the American Psychoanalytic Association,* 48:1055–1096.

Miller, J. (1985), How Kohut actually worked. In: *Progress in Self Psychology,* Vol. I, ed. A. Goldberg. New York: Guilford Press, pp. 13–30.

Nelson, K. (1986), *Event Knowledge.* Hillsdale, NJ: Lawrence Erlbaum Associates, Inc.

Renik, O. (1997), Reactions to "observing-participation, mutual enactment, and the new classical models" by I. Hirsch. *Contemp. Psychoanaly.,* 33:279–284.

Shane, M., Shane, E., & Gales, M. (1998), *Intimate Attachments: Toward a New Self Psychology.* New York: Guilford Press.

Slavin, M. & Kriegman, D. (1992), *The Adaptive Design of the Human Psyche.* New York: Guilford Press.

Slochower, J. (1996), *Holding and Psychoanalysis.* Hillsdale, NJ: The Analytic Press.

Stern, D. N. (1985), *The Interpersonal World of the Infant.* New York: Basic Books.

_____, Sander, L., Nahum, J., Harrison, A., Lyons-Ruth, K., Morgan, A., Bruschweiler-Stern, N., & Tronick, E. (1998), Non-interpretive mechanisms in psychoanalytic therapy: The "something more" than interpretation. *Int. J. Psycho-Anal.,* 79:903–921.

Stolorow, R., Brandchaft, B., & Atwood, G. (1987), *Psychoanalytic Treatment.* Hillsdale, NJ: The Analytic Press.

_____, Atwood, G., & Orange, D. (2002), *Worlds of Experience.* New York: Basic Books.

Tolpin, M. (2002), Doing psychoanalysis of normal development: Forward edge transferences. In: *Postmodern Self Psychology: Progress in Self Psychology,* Vol. 18, ed. A. Goldberg. Hillsdale, NJ: The Analytic Press, pp. 167–190.

Winnicott, D. (1965). *The Maturational Processes and the Facilitating Environment: Studies in the Theory of Emotional Development.* New York: International Universities Press.

250 West 57th Street, Suite 501
New York, NY 10019
fosshage@psychoanalysis.net

"The Strangest Remembrance": The Analyst's Intersubjective Negotiation of Desire: Commentary on Holly Levenkron, L.C.S.W.

BARBARA A. PIZER, ED.D., ABPP
STUART A. PIZER, PH.D., ABPP

In this commentary we emphasize that what Levenkron calls "the process wherein negotiating enactments becomes intersubjective relating" requires negotiation that is intrapsychic as well as relational and that it entails the analyst's internal negotiation between her transferences and her recognitions. We argue that the loss of paradoxical tension between transference and recognition is the breakdown of intersubjectivity. The analyst marooned in her own transference position will persist in negation of the other. We examine the sessions between Levenkron and Ali, noting the complementarity of their transferences, and trace the clinical process whereby analyst and patient recreate intersubjectivity in their relationship.

Barbara A. Pizer, Ed.D., ABPP is Supervising Analyst and Faculty, Massachusetts Institute for Psychoanalysis; Assistant Clinical Professor of Psychology, Harvard Medical School; Faculty, Program for Psychotherapy, The Cambridge Hospital; and Member, Board of Directors, International Association for Relational Psychoanalysis and Psychotherapy. She is a Contributing Editor of *Psychoanalytic Dialogues*.

Stuart A. Pizer, Ph.D., ABPP is Past-President, International Association for Relational Psychoanalysis and Psychotherapy; Past-President, Supervising Analyst and Faculty, Massachusetts Institute for Psychoanalysis; Assistant Clinical Professor of Psychology, Harvard Medical School; Faculty, Program for Psychotherapy, The Cambridge Hospital. He is a Contributing Editor of *Psychoanalytic Dialogues* and author of *Building Bridges: The Negotiation of Paradox in Psychoanalysis* (The Analytic Press, 1998).

HOLLY LEVENKRON HAS OFFERED US AN ARTICLE COURAGEOUS IN ITS candor and valuable in its sharing of the intimate intrasubjective and intersubjective process she experienced with Ali. In doing so, she has provided vivid illustration of the essential clinical phenomenon of ongoing breakdown and restoration of recognition between analyst and patient and the potential for an ultimately larger trajectory toward increasingly intimate and differentiated mutual recognition and growth. Levenkron[1] seeks to illustrate "the relationship among confrontation, enactment, and dissociation." She introduces her concept of "affective honesty" and emphasizes the intrinsic therapeutic action of intensely engaged, affectively charged enactments in the analytic dyad. "Specifically," she writes, "I am focusing on the process wherein negotiating enactments becomes intersubjective relating." In this discussion we will emphasize that enactments become intersubjective relating through a process of negotiation that is intrapsychic as well as relational and entailing the analyst's internal negotiation between her transferences and her recognitions. Loss of the paradoxical tension between transference and recognition is the breakdown of intersubjectivity. We persist in negation of the other when we are marooned in our own transference position. Holly's sessions with Ali beautifully illustrate the complementarity of their transferences based on maternal identifications and the clinical process whereby Holly and her patient recreate intersubjectivity between them.

Holly suggests that intersubjective space is "a construct that two people achieve through a collision of their realities," and that this collision may become intersubjective "if they each have to surrender 'some' of the hold they each had on their subjectivity in order to pay attention to the other person." As Benjamin (1988, 2000) has pointed out, enactments occur during breakdowns in the paradoxical tensions of intersubjectivity. That is, the person ceases to be able to hold in juxtaposition the recognition and negation of the other or, in Winnicottian terms, the object subjectively conceived and the object objectively perceived as existing separately out in the world. During breakdown and attendant enactments, there is an exchange of negations, the polarizations to which Holly refers and an exchange based in solipsistic subjectivity missing internal reflective functioning. Holly nicely

---

[1]Henceforth we will refer to Levenkron as Holly. Although surname is standard form for reference to an author, we believe that Holly suits the intimacy of the clinical vignettes under discussion. For stylistic consistency throughout, we will maintain the use of Levenkron's given name.

argues, and exemplifies, how such moments of enactment need not necessarily be signs of a treatment gone awry, a sovereignty of projective identifications, or a miring in analyst countertransference. Rather, her article offers a more normative view of enactment as the analytically lived struggle toward negotiation of breakdowns in the paradoxical tensions of true relatedness, the very stuff of the growth of the self in both parties. As Benjamin (1988) has written

> After all, breakdown of tension is as much a part of life as recreating it once more. The logic of paradox includes the acknowledgement that breakdown occurs. A sufficient ground for optimism is the contention that if breakdown is "built into" the psychic system, so is the possibility of renewing tension. If the denial of recognition does not become frozen into unmovable relationships, the play of power need not be hardened into domination. As the practice of psychoanalysis reveals, breakdown and renewal are constant possibilities: the crucial issue is finding the point at which breakdown occurs and the point at which it is possible to recreate tension and restore the condition of recognition [p. 223].

Holly's article takes us through such plays of power, their reciprocal deployment and calcification—what Holly calls "control operations"—and their negotiated release within the challenging dynamics of mutual enactment. Holly argues for "the idea that to whatever degree we give up our tight hold on our own subjectivity we increase the potential to validate the other person's subjectivity—while still retaining our own." We would suggest that it is not just "giving up a tight hold"; it's recognizing where in our own subjectivity a breakdown has occurred in the tension between subjectivization and recognition. This is not just a matter of being nimble, flexible, or supple but of facing down our own "blind spots" (McLaughlin, 1991), an act of self-recognition that reopens a space that has been occluded by our own activated transferences. We believe that Holly wishes to represent the process of negotiating enactments in the direction of intersubjectivity as something larger, for her, than insight into transferences and countertransferences. We agree that it feels that way experientially. And yet we remain impressed with the wisdom in McLaughlin's (1991) writings on enactment and propose that his perspective usefully augments Holly's. Holly asserts that "it bears repeating that during the evolution of every treatment—each person tries to change the other person in terms of conscious and unconscious agendas on each of their parts, and to one degree or another, the need to change the other person (as in most relationships) is often opposed and fails to be met.... The challenge is in changing—in allowing the interaction to shape us." Compare this with McLaughlin (1991):

> [W]hether analyst or patient, our deepest hopes for what we may find the world to be, as well as our worst fears of what it will be, reflect our transference expectancies as shaped by our developmental past. We busy ourselves through life with words and actions aimed at obtaining some response in self and other, in keeping with these expectancies [p. 599].

And, as McLaughlin further declares

> ... the transference ghosts of the past are never entirely laid to rest. In the intensity of new work with qualities unique and not yet known, they return in fresh shape to revive shades of significance I had long forgotten I knew. Enactments are my expectable lot [p. 613].

Putting together McLaughlin's concept of the analyst's transference blind spots and Benjamin's ideas about the natural inevitability of breakdown and reestablishment of the tensions of recognition, we would elaborate on a statement of Holly's. She asserts, "Moving toward relatedness is a negotiation, but it isn't about winning; it's about changing our experience to get closer to what we want while staying related to the other person." We agree. But what is "changing our experience"? And how does it relate to the process, at the center of Holly's interest, "wherein negotiating enactments becomes intersubjective relating"? We suggest that "changing our experience" involves an act of reflection or a shift in perspective on our own transferences. As S. Pizer (1992, 1998) has elsewhere written, negotiation is not simply deal making or consensus building. It is a multileveled bridging of internal, or intrapsychic, as well as relational paradoxes. These paradoxes include transference and "real," old and new, and who at any moment in the analytic dyad is doing what to whom. Perhaps Holly means to imply all of this in her reference to "changing our experience." We believe that the give-and-take of analytic negotiation Holly depicts also makes important operative use of Bromberg's (1998) postulate, which captures another essential paradox. Bromberg proposes that "the human personality possesses

the extraordinary capacity to negotiate stability and change simultaneously, and it will do so under the right relational conditions—conditions
that preserve every patient's necessary illusion that 'he can stay the same
while changing'" (p. 209). Bromberg views resistance as the enacted communication of a patient's struggle to straddle the paradoxes of self-continuity and change in the analytic process. We might declare that the same
holds true for the analyst! And this inherent capacity to stay the same while
changing is born of the intrinsic human need for relatedness held in paradoxical juxtaposition with the intrinsic need for intrapsychic privacy, autonomy, and self-continuity. This is why, as S. Pizer (1998) wrote, analyst
and patient are recurrently saying to each other, "No, you can't make this of
me. But you can make that of me" (p. 3). Or, as Holly puts it, "each person
tries to change the other person in terms of conscious and unconscious
agendas on each of their parts, and to one degree or another, the need to
change the other person … is often opposed and fails to be met." And recall
McLaughlin's apt observation that "we busy ourselves through life with
words and actions aimed at obtaining some response in self and other, in
keeping with … expectancies [shaped by our developmental past]." Holly's
case is a beautiful illustration of the intrinsic need for human relatedness.
She provides for us the clinical terrain of certain interactions whose subjective components—for both Ali and Holly—include a developmental past,
an intrapsychic history, as well as an ongoing interpersonal negotiation.
And, as Benjamin has articulated for us, intersubjectivity is located in *the
tension of intrapsychic and interpersonal held in conjunction.*

Intersubjectivity is not a culminative or static state of grace or psychic
merger. Rather it is the sustained tension between the hold of the
intrapsychic and the draw of human relatedness. The tension of intersubjectivity can be created only as each person extricates herself from
some enmeshment in relation to her own intrapsychic objects—that is,
her transferences. We are always bridging outwardly to the other, and yet
we are always also not bridging to the other as we bridge inwardly to the
intrapsychic center of object–relational representation and fantasy within
ourselves—or, in Bromberg's terms, we are always staying the same
while changing. This sustained tension is the ongoing negotiation of
intersubjectivity. It reflects the basic human need to relate and to negotiate relatedness while holding onto selfhood, or separate subjectivity. And
this negotiation always bridges between finding the other outside (or recognition) and a conscription of the other to represent the object of desire
and also the opposing side of internal splits, repetitions of old (and often

traumatizing) object ties, the reversible complementarity of intrapsychic enmeshments and identifications—in short, our transferences.

Thus, we would say that "moving toward relatedness" is an *intrapsychic* and *interpersonal* negotiation, but it isn't about winning; it's about *becoming aware of our transferences in the midst of the interpersonal experience to get closer to who we are and where we're coming from* as well as what we want, while staying related to the other person. In the immediacy of analytic enactments, affect and disclosure, and also aspects of what Holly calls our "realness," are being negotiated between two subjectivities—a squiggling toward coconstructed emergent shapes of being, feeling, remembering, and relating. And we believe that the clinical relationship between enactment and emergent intersubjectivity— the focus of Holly's paper—involves the analyst's internal negotiation of some awareness of his or her self relocated as a participant within the transference–countertransference matrix. We must allow the patient to colonize our mind, as Fonagy (quoted in Coates, 1998) put it, and then refind our own bearings while maintaining a bridge to what has been made of us in the force field of interactive subjectivities. Sandler (1976) was referring to a related process when he wrote about the analyst's becoming aware of tacit role-responsiveness; and Symington (1983) described the process in terms of the analyst's act of freedom in extricating from embeddedness in a "corporate identity" with the patient. Bromberg (1998) emphasizes the analyst's awakening from a dissociative state reciprocal to disavowed and dissociated aspects of the patient that have found inclusion in the analytic relationship through enactment. Holly underscores a position very much in line with Fonagy, Sandler, Symington, and Bromberg, as well as Davies. She writes

As patient and analyst associate and dissociate (Davies, 1998) to each other's psychic contents—there are inevitable shifts in their respective realities that can move the relationship in any number of directions. In particular, I believe it is through the expansion of enactments that dissociated and conflicted mental contents are brought forward into awareness.

We would suggest, in concert with McLaughlin's perspective, that the analyst should also be associating to her own psychic contents and, further, that it is through a deeper awareness of the analyst's own transferences embedded in unfolding enactments that "dissociated and conflicted mental content are brought forward into awareness." We think that this readiness to face ourselves down in the thick of mutual enactment defines what Holly calls "affective honesty." That is, we are affectively honest when we are both affectively engaged and also accountable for our own intrasubjective wellsprings that have been activated within the unfolding analytic encounter. Holly says it well when she declares that "the craft within this field lies in calling on something in us to navigate [mutual] influences—not as technique in a contrived prescripted way—but by contacting a part of ourselves that can own—either to ourselves or out loud to our patient—what it is we are doing in the interaction." It is just here that we may succeed for the moment in negotiating a movement from "doer" and "done to" toward a more complex and paradoxical mutual recognition.

Holly's three clinical vignettes illustrate this passage very well. Before turning our attention to this rich clinical material, we want to reemphasize that the outflow into analytic space of enactive intensities from the deep recesses of the analyst's mind cannot be assumed to represent a moment of clinical incompetence or psychic incontinence but rather a naturally occurring and recurring component of the oscillating positions of intersubjectivity. Russell (1975) pointed out that each treatment will have its "crunches," and that in the moment of crunch the question of "is this you or is it me" is impossible to answer. The crunch is about how each party is both "doer" and "done to," reflective functioning has lapsed, potential space is collapsed, and there is a breakdown in recognition of self or other beyond the current concrete terms of enactment. Benjamin (2000) has addressed this issue recently in a way that we think is quite germane to our consideration of Holly's intrapsychic struggle within the intersubjective space she shared with Ali. Benjamin writes

> Only by enlisting the analyst's subjectivity to play the opposing part in the split can the patient hope to reveal certain parts of self. From a relational point of view, *enactment is inevitable because only a two-person dynamic can make visible and compelling the thing needing to be spoken,* which arose in a two person dynamic.... Thus, rather than simply revealing the analyst's subjectivity or personhood, the analyst's disclosure represents the necessary component in the two-person dynamic, "the subjugating third," in which the analyst allows his personal history to assume a form dictated by the relationship [pp. 52–53].

Holding this perspective in mind, let's now turn our attention to the three sessions between Holly and Ali as we seek to articulate "the point at which breakdown occurs and the point at which it is possible to recreate tension and restore the condition of recognition" (Benjamin, 2000). Benefiting from Holly's generosity in presenting the clinical material, we are in the privileged position of moving either forward in time or backward in time through the three sessions. We begin with a key moment in session three, in which Holly reports having "the strangest remembrance." Holly recalls that, as her own mother was dying, Holly was not allowed her own feelings ("she would not let me cry") and she was not protected from her terrors. Holly was thus caught up in the enormity of an experience in which she could not find or declare her separate subjectivity in relation to the other. And it was only after Holly found that she could survive that she accessed her wistfulness at the missed opportunity for intersubjective sharing with her mother and a more loving separation. It strikes us that, at this moment of self-recognition during her session with Ali, Holly dramatically climbs out of her enactment of breakdown and restores the tension at the heart of intersubjectivity. We suggest that these three sessions prove to be intimately interlocking expressions of the theme of separation. Ali and Holly are each identified with their intrapsychic mothers and thereby installed in a state of reversible complementarity. We will particularly focus on Holly's gallant intrasubjective and intersubjective work to emerge from this enactment. Let us also state that what Ali brings out in Holly may not be the fullness of who Holly's mother was for Holly but, specifically, Holly's mother for Holly in the moment of her mother's dying—in particular, her intrapsychic defensive denial and her relational withdrawal. So that, when we refer to Holly as relating from the intrapsychic position of her mother, bear in mind that we mean Holly's mother as we imagine Holly represented her internally in the experience of her dying.

Now let's visit session one and move forward in time through the process between Holly and Ali. Holly walks upstairs ahead of Ali, and Ali fixes upon Holly's legs and then, in the session, fixes upon Holly in a seductive, mocking, and space-collapsing way. She shakes her shaming index finger, as if to say "now, now—you bad girl." Holly pulls back, asking herself, "Was I, in fact, aroused?" Ali feels foreign to her, as if assuming a relationship that Holly is not offering. And Holly concludes, "we both had to be deprived."

When Ali says to Holly, "you knew I would look at your legs. Now, Holly," she is certainly conjuring an eroticized, flirtatiously "doer–done to" relationship between them that rattles Holly. But we will conjecture here that, within the deep matrix of interlocking maternal transferences, Ali is saying to Holly "You *are* what I make of you." Hence, frightening and repellant feeling for Holly entails her being in Ali's position in relation to Ali's enmeshing mother. Whereas Ali's internal mother enmeshes, Holly's internal mother withdraws. In either case, the person is left unrecognized as a separate person—or, paraphrasing Holly, "we both had to be deprived." When Holly reports that Ali shakes her finger "as if to say 'now, now—you bad girl'," Holly's narrative use of an unreflective "as if" suggests Holly's transference fantasy. At that moment, Holly is Holly in relation to her own mother (feeling her own affective reality to be invalidated); she is also her own mother in relation to Holly (rejecting an unwelcome feeling); and she is Ali in relation to Ali's mother (whom Ali is enacting in her demand for merger). When Holly asks herself, "Was I aroused?" (was I feeling something I shouldn't?), it is an indication that she has indeed been "done to," undone by Ali, or Ali's mother, or, in the intrapsychic realm, her own mother. Holly writes that "here Ali was assuming a relationship I was not offering." We suggest that this refers not only to sexual titillation but to a relationship based on sameness and enmeshment—that is, "you are exactly and only what I make of you"—and not an intimacy in which self and other exist in a shared space. Holly, who values the experience of liking another and interacting in an honest and passionate way, struggles to find how to be analytically useful "in the storm of my countertransference." She is stymied by what she terms Ali's "distancing and assuming behavior." As we read it, *Holly* was distancing from Ali's *assuming* behavior. Ali's distancing behavior *follows* from this because Ali is then scolding Holly for distancing (as Holly's mother distanced from Holly's desires for emotional connection). Ali, in her scolding, is—for Holly—like Holly's mother rebuking Holly's wish for a real relational connection. And Ali cannot yet see the repellant nature of her scolding because, intrapsychically, she is unseparated from her own mother who assumed and required merger.

Holly reports that *"from deep within the experience of these tensions I recall feeling very bad for wanting to reject Ali."* Holly does not want to be like her own mother, rejecting the desire of the other. Just as this may be one step out of an unconscious (or dissociated) identification with the affectively withdrawn mother, Holly may also be accessing some inkling of what her own mother could have felt as she distanced emotionally from her daughter while managing her own existential dread. Holly comes to "understand" Ali's "wish and fantasy that I desire her to desire me." Ali's wish is also Holly's wish, with Ali and with mother: that the other would welcome my desire and my feelings, that the relationship would accommodate an intimate sharing of affective honesty. Holly speaks from her position "stuck between my own boundaries and Ali's pain," saying you can't get from a relationship what you want by demanding. Unlike her mother, who persisted in denying her own death, Holly was able to confront her own wishes for "release" from Ali's demands and to convey this message in a way that Ali could hear, thus sponsoring an emergent two-person process. Ali cries, and Holly feels shaken. Holly is taking steps to find her way out of the entrenched complementarity of maternal identifications. She can now register Ali's statement of a fear of abandonment as a note of negotiation—as, indeed, it seems to be. In naming her feeling, Ali in that moment conjures a "reflective third" to represent her feeling; and this contrasts with her pattern of enacting the "subjugating third" of coercing merger. But in the process of working through, there is more to come.

In session two, Holly's short notice announcement of her departure for a week incites in Ali anger and envy. In the transference, Ali asserts her conviction that wonderful things are about to happen to Holly. For Holly, the moment is suffocating. Holly tells us that "with tears welling in my eyes … all I was in touch with was a strong wish for her to stop torturing me." We might at this moment describe Ali's impact on Holly with the words used later, in session three, to describe Holly's mother: "She would not even consider that I needed to be protected in any way." Holly finds herself struggling with "a powerful urge to tell her every bad thing that ever happened to me, that is, just how hard my life had really been and certainly how hard it was at that time." Once again, Holly's mind is being colonized by Ali—or, more accurately, by Ali's mother within Ali—as Ali's envious attack renders her state when threatened with loss. And once again Holly is moved to declare "I have my feelings too!" Here, again, she is Ali in relation to Ali's mother as well as herself in relation to her own mother. Caught in breakdown, Holly insists in an angry tone, "Right now this is all I can give you. Next week that may change." Holly reports to us that, for her, saying this "meant I was separate." This may remind us of Holly's later statement in relation to her mother's dying, that "when I saw that I could survive"—that is, when Holly could be separate from psychic colonization by the unspeakable—she was able to move out of the torture of her terror to the more reflective wish that she "could have shared more with her."

We might conjecture here that the part of the enactment in session two that still remains within Holly's transference is reflected in "Nondisclosure as a Substitute for Confrontation." Holly rationalizes this technical choice with the thought that "I was protecting her from feeling guilty for attacking" and she was also protecting herself from protracted sadistic pummeling. Although Holly also recognizes that "nondisclosure was a clear expression of my subjectivity" and that she wants to break free of the bonds of enslavement. From what? Holly's enactment may include, in an identification with the manner of her mother's dying, the message that "I am going away, but I'm not offering you access to what is going on inside me." To be left in the absence of affective sharing can be a negation. What Holly does come closer to understanding is that her own subjectivity "included my own wishes to interact in an honest, passionate way with another human being, as well as the right to get angry when my boundaries were intruded on." Holly distinguishes this from a "countertransference experience," seeing it as something broader, more encompassing, more enlisting of the total relationship as a "third party." And, indeed, we believe Holly is describing, and bringing into conceptualization, a compelling example of just what Benjamin meant when she asserted that "rather than simply revealing the analyst's subjectivity or personhood, the analyst's disclosure [or, in this case, enactment of nondisclosure] represents the necessary component in the two-person dynamic, 'the subjugating third', in which the analyst allows his personal history to assume a form dictated by the relationship."

Holly is moving out of the transference–countertransference enactment in which reciprocal power plays and control operations fight negation with negation. Locating her own subjectivity within the confines of "the subjugating third," Holly registers that "it was imperative to *have the choice* of consciously speaking with my patient directly about my personal experience of her." Like freeing herself from her terror over the enforced denial of her mother's dying, Holly was free to make choices with Ali. She didn't have to agree with her mother's "reality" (of denial) and she doesn't have to agree with Ali's "reality" of merger and defensive assaults. With a "dramatic shift," Holly makes creative use of her own history, affirming that "I wanted to strike a balance between protecting her (recognizing her vulnerability) and protecting myself, so that her subjectivity did not do violence to me; along with maintaining an open channel to express my point of view." We are reminded of how B. Pizer defines intimacy: not an agreement, not a knowing of every detail about another's process and thoughts, but "the ability to be one's self in the presence of another." The hope entering the collapsed space between Holly and Ali, opening toward a more capacious intersubjective space, lies in the paradox that these two women, who deeply share the feeling that they had to take care of their mothers by not having their own separate feelings, can now begin to join together in feeling differently in each other's presence.

And now we are at session three. As Holly tells us, "our patients ... make us aware of what we have dissociated." In this session, Holly comes to recognize how deeply Ali worries about Holly's heart. Ali begins prompting Holly to emerge from her denial by exclaiming, "Why can't I just come in and have a feeling.... It's all right for you to say whatever you want, so why not me. Why are you getting so bent out of shape, Holly?" Not yet able to attend to this confrontation, Holly is once again feeling suffocated by Ali's raw demands. In this ensuing crunch, Holly (surmounting inhibition) asserts that "this could destroy this therapy.... I don't want that to happen—so help me out here." And Ali is able to own that she is blinded by her need to merge with Holly. And Holly becomes able to ask, "do you feel that my being separate means you would be alone forever?" In this single query, Holly gathers up the question she might also address to herself, joining the affective meanings in all three sessions—indeed, the question that we all may well ask ourselves in the face of the death of a loved one or when contemplating a marital separation. That is, in relation to (1) desiring to be desired and (2) separation from a husband and (3) a mother's death, "do you feel that ... being separate means you would be alone forever?"

And so Holly arrives with Ali at a clear intersubjective moment that recreates the paradoxical tension of separation and connection and restores the condition of mutual recognition. Holly makes a statement that deeply recognizes both Ali and herself. She says, "I didn't think anyone ever showed you that you can be safe even if you were separate." And Holly asks Ali, "if my going in for surgery left her feeling that I would die and leave her unprotected." Ali begins to cry. And Holly reports that "now I was able to tell her I hadn't realized how frightening that must have been for her." In an exchange of reparations and personal acknowledgments, and a spirit of mutual receptiveness and mutual survival, Holly says she is sorry not to have understood how scared Ali was of losing her but is also able to note how Ali's anger had impeded the evolution of closeness. And Ali is able to admit her own difficulty sustaining connection. In this intersubjective atmosphere, Holly experiences that "something had shifted in me" and she becomes "aware of wanting to act on my interest in being more open." Holly tells Ali what neither of their mothers had been able to say to their daughters, that they would both be OK. We might say that Holly stands now in a space separate from her de-

priving maternal identification and, from her heart, says what she had desired her dying mother to say to her. And here Holly receives her "strangest remembrance," defining the intersubjective moment in which Holly
climbed out of the enactment and negotiated her own internal recognition
of a vital transference "blind spot." And, unlike her own mother, Holly
doesn't deny death anymore.

Holly and Ali, no longer impelled to deny the haunting presence of a
mother's (or an analyst–mother's) mortality, can now sustain a connection
while speaking about differentiation and negotiate the experience of separation "in a loving way." To us, this represents the ongoing negotiation of
the paradoxes of intersubjectivity, forever incomplete in the analytic
duet—as in any living relationship.

REFERENCES

Benjamin, J. (1988), *The Bonds of Love.* New York: Pantheon Books.
_____ (2000), Intersubjective distinctions: Subjects and persons, recognitions and break-
    downs: Commentary on paper by Gerhardt, Sweetnam, and Borton. *Psychoanal. Dial.,*
    10:43–55.
Bromberg, P. (1998), *Standing in the Spaces: Essays on Clinical Process, Trauma & Disso-
    ciation.* Hillsdale, NJ: The Analytic Press.
Coates, S. W. (1998), Having a mind of one's own and holding the other in mind: Commen-
    tary on paper by Peter Fonagy and Mary Target. *Psychoanal. Dial.,* 8:115–148.
Davies, J. M. (1998), Multiple perspectives on multiplicity. *Psychoanal. Dial.,* 8:195–206.
McLaughlin, J. (1991), Clinical and theoretical aspects of enactments in the psychoanalytic
    situation. *J. Amer. Psychoanal. Assn.,* 39:595–614.
Pizer, S. A. (1992), The negotiation of paradox in the analytic process. *Psychoanal. Dial.,*
    2:215–240.
_____ (1998), *Building Bridges: The Negotiation of Paradox in Psychoanalysis.* Hillsdale,
    NJ: The Analytic Press.
Russell, P. (1975), The theory of the crunch. Unpublished manuscript.
Sandler, J. (1976), Countertransference and role-responsiveness. *Internat. Rev. Psy-
    cho-Anal.,* 3:43–47.
Symington, N. (1983), The analyst's act of freedom as agent of therapeutic change.
    Internat. Rev. Psycho-Anal., 10:283–291.

152 Brattle Street
Cambridge, MA 02138
bapizer@comcast.net

Discussion of Holly Levenkron's "Love (and Hate) With the Proper Stranger"

OWEN RENIK, M.D.

> I agree with Holly Levenkron that the value of an intersubjective perspective is pragmatic: It directs the analyst toward more effective technique. Also, I agree with her view that a successful analytic process is a negotiation between analyst and patient. However, I question Levenkron's idea that the analyst must loosen her hold on her own subjectivity in order for the negotiation to proceed. An analyst cannot and need not diminish her subjectivity. Rather, what is required for clinical analytic work to unfold is that the analyst include the patient within the analyst's subjectivity—or, in other words, that the analyst come to love the patient.

THE MEDIUM IS THE MESSAGE IN HOLLY'S ARTICLE. HER ACCOUNT OF her analytic work with Ali presents us with Holly's own affectively charged experience of clinical events so that we can interact with it. The method she uses to establish a dialogue with her readers is the same method Holly uses to establish a dialogue with her patient in the treatment setting. The aim in both instances is to optimize a productive intersubjective exchange.

Holly makes the very important point that the value of acknowledging the intersubjectivity of the clinical analytic encounter does not have to do with authenticity per se. Acknowledging the intersubjectivity of the clinical encounter is valuable because it directs us to more effective analytic technique. Intersubjective interaction is, as Holly puts it, "the most clini-

Owen Renik, M.D. is a Supervising and Training Analyst at the San Francisco Psychoanalytic Institute; and a Clinical Professor of Psychiatry at the University of California at San Francisco

cally powerful dimension of the analytic process." It forces each person to bring something new into the situation, Holly tells us. In saying this, she implicitly underlines the crucial understanding that every successful psychoanalysis is at heart a learning process. Learning is facilitated when the analyst proceeds with an acceptance of her irreducible subjectivity in mind. Holly is making a pragmatic, rather than a political, argument for a clinical approach informed by awareness of the intersubjectivity of the clinical psychoanalytic encounter.

I am very much in accord with Holly's view, following Stuart Pizer's work, that successful psychoanalysis is a negotiation. One place that I might slightly revise Holly's conceptualization of the negotiation is where she says that what is required of the analyst is to "give up her tight hold on her own subjectivity." To my mind, it is neither possible nor required that the analyst relinquish her own subjectivity to any extent at all. Of course, as Holly's clinical report illustrates very well, a successful psychoanalytic negotiation does demand of the analyst that she take serious account of the patient's point of view—which may be very different from her own point of view, even threatening to it. But I would not describe this evolution as the analyst loosening her hold on her own subjectivity. Rather, I would describe it as the analyst expanding her own subjectivity to include within it the patient's subjectivity, as best she understands it. I would describe what is required, in other words, as the analyst coming to love the patient. It seems to me that the whole subject of the analyst's love for the patient as a sine qua non for effective clinical work is one that we are just beginning to explore.

I think Holly's emphasis on the uniqueness of the communication within each psychoanalytic couple is all important. It reminds us of what it is easy to lose sight of in the heat of the clinical moment: that all truths arrived at in the treatment setting—the old truths that are "discovered" as well as the newly "constructed" truths that replace old truths—are cocreated by analyst and patient and therefore specific to that particular pair. This is not to say, of course, that what an individual learns from a particular psychoanalytic interaction cannot be generalized to other interpersonal interactions. If generalization were not possible, clinical psychoanalysis could confer no therapeutic benefit to the patient. Nonetheless, Holly's emphasis on the uniqueness of the clinical analytic dialogue directs us to a fuller appreciation of the intersubjectivity of our cocreations and helps us guard against idealization of them—both in our clinical work and in our communication with colleagues about our clinical work.

I must say that I have never found spatial metaphors of great help in discussing these matters. I confess to wincing a bit when I read Holly's reference to "the domain of intersubjective space." Frankly, I don't know what that means; and when a colleague speaks to me about some aspect of psychotherapy as a "space," I usually feel invited to share a hyperintellectual escape from the nitty gritty of analyst–patient interactions. Happily, however, Holly is issuing no such invitation. Quite the opposite, as we soon find out when we read her candid, down to earth descriptions of what happened between her and Ali and how they each felt about what happened.

A related theoretical question concerns the concept of enactment. How, exactly, does it help us to think about enactment in the treatment setting? It is my view, as Holly mentions, that using the term enactment to denote a discrete, identifiable clinical moment is misguided and misleading. The assumption is that some clinical events, enactments, express unconscious motivations of patient and/or analyst—corresponding to unconscious fantasies of analyst and/or patient—while other clinical events do not or do so to a lesser extent. The truth is, however, that every clinical event expresses the unconscious motivations of the participants and corresponds to their unconscious fantasies somehow or other; and since the motivations and fantasies in question are unconscious, the participants are not able to assess the nature and the extent of the expression and correspondence. Occasionally, they catch a retrospective glimpse of a tiny fraction of what is ongoing every minute of the time.

Furthermore, even if we use the term enactment to denote an ongoing aspect of all clinical events, the concept is problematic and of questionable value. Originally, Freud formulated the concept of acting out based on his hydraulic model of the mind in which impulses sought motor discharge but could be blocked and redirected. It was Freud's idea that motor discharge of psychic impulses had to be prevented in order to force the impulses to reverse their direction and stimulate the sensory apparatus from within, creating thoughts that could then be analyzed. Thus, Freud thought that fantasies and their constituent motivations, if acted out, would not be available for analysis. As the progress of neural science and accumulating psychoanalytic experience, rendered Freud's original model of the mind obsolete, his concept of acting out became more difficult to justify. Enactment, a fuzzier, less theoretically specific term, replaced acting out as the preferred usage. But in fact enactment is essentially a euphemism for acting out. Both derive from the same (erroneous) assumption that thought and motor action are mutually exclusive alternatives. If we look carefully at Holly's instructive account and discussion of her therapy with Ali, I think we find that there is nothing described that depends on the concept of enactment. Holly could have done just as well without it.

The problem is compounded when Holly refers to the "working through of enactments" in successful psychoanalysis. What does "working through" mean here? Surely, Holly is not referring to the traditional psychoanalytic concept of working through, which was an ill-defined, even mysterious, process thought to occur during the often observed lag between "correct analytic work" and the appearance of therapeutic benefit! Actually, if Holly is looking for a term to use when speaking of the clinical events that form the substrate of a therapeutically successful psychoanalysis, I think she might just as well stick with her original emphasis on negotiation and speak of the negotiation of corrective emotional experiences between analyst and patient. It seems to me that the contributions of Alexander and French (1946), who coined the term corrective emotional experience, and Weiss and Sampson (1998) who elaborated a theory of clinical analysis based on it, remain useful. We may question the technical approaches that those authors recommend as being presumptuous or contrived in certain respects, but that in no way invalidates their conceptions of how learning takes place in a successful clinical psychoanalysis. If we do not speak of "enactment," or of "the working through of enactments" but say instead that Holly and Ali managed, between them, to negotiate a number of crucial emotional experiences that helped Ali correct certain maladaptive expectations and ways of coping with those expectations, will we lose anything?

Holly's case report is an illustrative example, par excellence, of how there are many ways through the woods and of how ignoble motivations on an analyst's part often play a decisive role in a successful clinical psychoanalytic process. By sharing with us her report of a familiarly confusing treatment experience, conducted many times on a trial and error basis, she makes her point. I will only elaborate a very little bit by focusing on a detail in Holly's case report that struck me as interesting.

I was brought up short when I realized that Holly was seeing Ali on the couch! Given that the interaction between Holly and Ali, which began the sequence that Holly found so significant concerned Ali's accusation that Holly wanted to be looked at, I wondered how it was that Holly's positioning herself out of Ali's view during most of their time together did not come up as a relevant matter for discussion between them. Even more important, I wondered why Holly chose to use the couch at all in her treatment of Ali. Originally, Freud was quite frank about sitting behind the patient because he preferred not to be scrutinized. Later, what began as a candidly self-protective preference on Freud's part came to be rationalized as being necessary for the patient's welfare: the analyst stayed outside the patient's field of vision so that the patient could free associate with minimum distraction. But, of course, that rationalization pertains to a conception of treatment based on a one-person psychology—that the patient projects onto a screen that is kept as blank as possible—a conception that is entirely opposite to the intersubjectivist one that Holly advocates. From an intersubjectivist perspective, the analyst, rather than trying to remain anonymous, tries to make herself maximally available to be known by the patient (to use Ken Frank's, 1997, excellent phrase). Remaining invisible, seated upright above a reclining patient, would seem to be the very last thing Holly would want to do.

Similarly, I did not understand Holly's explanation about why she refused to tell Ali that the sudden cancellation was necessary because Holly was taking a week off to deal with the dissolution of her marriage. I certainly agree that it is not a good idea for an analyst to automatically and indiscriminately accommodate a patient's curiosity. And I agree that it can be very useful for an analyst to confront a patient with the analyst's sense of entitlement to certain self-interested motivations. But in those instances, it is of the utmost importance that the analyst be honest about being self-interested and not try to pass off her choice as being for the patient's benefit. It seemed to me that it might have been very helpful for Ali to know that Holly's life had some important problem areas, especially given Ali's problematic, recalcitrant envy of Holly. Therefore, I could not see any therapeutically oriented reason for Holly to decline to disclose the purpose of her week off. Obviously, Holly was dealing with a difficult and distressing personal situation, and I could well imagine that Holly might not feel comfortable talking to Ali about it; however, in that case, why didn't Holly explain that she preferred, for reasons of her own comfort, to keep the reason for her sudden absence private? As it was, in her explanations to Ali and to the reader, Holly seems to be invoking the virtues of selective analytic anonymity; and I find her position on the matter inconsistent with her conception of the way treatment works and with the treatment approach she advocates in general. The effect on Ali of Holly's refusal to disclose the reason for her sudden absence appears to have been to perpetuate Ali's idealization of Holly. Holly avoided the possibility of being perceived as imperfect: instead of learning that Holly's marriage was coming to an end, Ali could continue to believe that Holly and her husband were going off on some marvelous vacation, the details of which Holly didn't want to tell her.

I have the impression that covert elements of a traditionally authoritarian analytic stance remained defensively active in Holly's way of dealing with Ali, despite Holly's intention to adopt a "relational" approach. I think Holly is aware of this when she describes her difficulty avoiding power struggles with Ali. Power was surely the central matter about which they negotiated. Even at the beginning, when Ali suggested that Holly preceded her up the stairs to show off her legs and Holly denied it, the important issue was power, not sexual arousal. To my mind, there was a measure of truth in Ali's complaint that Holly was "a controlling monster." Ali brought a lively capacity for envy with her a priori, but certain elements of Holly's approach exacerbated Ali's envy unnecessarily. How analyst and patient found their way out of this impasse is the instructive story of Holly's successful analysis with Ali. It is a pertinent account of what Holly terms an intersubjective exchange. It is also an account of how Holly and Ali negotiated a series of emotional experiences from which Ali (and Holly as well, though that was an elective bonus) learned some crucial lessons—many of them never explicitly identified and examined.

I'm grateful to Holly for sharing the story with us, giving us the possibility of expanding our clinical awareness by interacting with her clinical experience—including what some might call her errors. We do well to remember, though, that so-called errors are part of every successful treatment. In clinical analysis, it is not the analyst's job to be right all the time; the analyst's job is to facilitate a productive learning process for the patient. Similarly, with respect to an article published in an analytic journal, it is not the author's job to be right all the time; the author's job is to stimulate a productive learning process for the reader. In my judgment, Holly can count both her analysis with Ali and the article she wrote about that analysis jobs well done.

REFERENCES

Alexander, F. and French, T. (1946) *Psychoanalytic Therapy: Principles and Applications.* New York: Ronald Press

Frank, K. (1997) The role of the analyst's inadvertent self-revelations. *Psychoanalytic Dialogues*, 7:281–314.

Weiss, J. (1998) Unconscious plan and unconscious conflict. *Phychoanalytic Dialogues*, 8:443–447.

388 Market St. Ste. 1010
San Francisco, CA 94111
Odrenik@aol.com

Affective Honesty and Compassion Come in Many Forms: Discussion of "Love (and Hate) With the Proper Stranger: Affective Honesty and Enactment," by Holly Levenkron, L.I.C.S.W.

MALCOLM OWEN SLAVIN, PH.D.

Holly Levenkron's work with her patient, Ali, beautifully illustrates one way that a creative analyst makes superb use of her own experience to communicate and negotiate with great affective honesty. Holly's analytic style emphasizes the effective use of a particular kind of self-disclosure and a way of thinking about intersubjectivity and enactment associated with the contemporary Relational movement. Yet, it may be Holly's personal willingness to allow the analytic relationship to profoundly destabilize and influence her that most engages Ali in their work.

An imaginary analytic scenario is described with an analyst, Dr. X, who like Holly is destabilized by Ali but whose thinking about intersubjectivity and enactment emphasizes an empathic immersion in Ali's experience of the analytic relationship. In contrast to Holly, Dr. X focuses primarily on grasping and interpreting the adaptive strivings that animate Ali's differently organized subjective world.

The underlying capacity to acknowledge and use the analyst's own version of the patient's issues may also characterize analyses such as that of the

Malcolm Owen Slavin, Ph.D. is a founder, supervising analyst, and chair of the postgraduate fellowship program at the Massachusetts Institute for Psychoanalysis (MIP). He is a Contributing Editor for *Psychoanalytic Dialogues* and is on the Editorial Board of the *International Journal for the Psychology of the Self*. His book *The Adaptive Design of the Human Psyche: Psychoanalysis, Evolutionary Biology and the Therapeutic Process* (written with Daniel Kriegman) was published by Guilford Press in 1992.

hypothetical Dr. X—in style that are more explicitly "interpretive" (less confrontative) than Holly's work. These two contrasting approaches highlight the wide range of ways to think about intersubjectivity, enactment, and affective honesty in the analytic process.

ONE OF THE MOST INTERESTING AND VALUABLE THINGS THAT HAS happened to me in recent years is to have the opportunity to supervise a great many analyses both at my own institute and at other training programs around the country. Observing and playing a part in so many intimate analytic relationships—so many unfolding lives—has affirmed some of my deepest beliefs about the *mutuality of influence* in a fruitful analysis, and *disconfirmed*—or called into question—many of the notions I've held about *how* the process of analytic influence needs to take place.

Some of the themes that emerge in any productive analysis—the human, existential challenges faced, the mutual quality of the struggle, the reciprocal nature of change, seem *virtually universal*. Conversely, universal notions of analytic technique—that is, prescriptive notions (mine or anyone's) about how analysts *should* behave—usually dissolve in the face of the almost infinitely variable forms that emerge in the lived, creative realities of different analytic couples. I am not sure if, unlike Tolstoy's "unhappy families," failed analyses turn out to be more monotonously alike than successful ones. I am, however, increasingly confident that fruitful analyses ultimately rely on the capacity of each analytic couple to construct unique, creative solutions to their own versions of the universal, adaptive challenges of the analytic crunch (Russell, unpublished). In short, happy analyses seem to turn out to be almost endlessly, unpredictably, varied.

Affective Honesty, Compassion, and the Patient's Impact on the Analyst

Holly Levenkron's beautifully written narrative of her relationship and heartfelt, inventive work with Ali is clearly one of those creatively unfolding analyses. As such, I read it primarily as the story of how Holly experiences, grows, and communicates around several major conflicts that emerge in their relationship. Holly wrestles with what feels to her like Ali's violation of, or misreading of, Holly's subjectivity (her desires, her marriage, even her bodily vulnerability, and, ultimately, her mortality). Holly does not squeeze the experience of those subjective clashes into any of the easily available technical or theoretical categories that can sometimes give us the illusion of understanding and correctly responding—at the expense of remaining painfully, intimately present with our patients. Her patient, Ali, appears to feel the deep, personal giving that this entails. Although we don't hear its dénouement, or how the patient's life actually changes, Ali does seem to open herself more fully to Holly and, as time goes by, to being influenced by the analytic process.

What I am describing about Holly's approach is, in outline, the kind of responsiveness that I think Holly refers to when she speaks of "affective honesty." I am with her in spades so far as she emphasizes and promotes this central aspect of the analyst's struggle for self-awareness and genuineness in communicating with her patient. Indeed, as I see it, Holly paints an extraordinarily vivid picture of the universal, reciprocal, emotional opening up that, in my view, is implicitly called for by the patient in many intersubjective clashes in analytic relationships.

It is, however, a little harder for me to feel as fully in agreement with Holly when she couples her superb grasp of the importance of "affective honesty" with what can be read as (1) her tendency to equate a certain type of *confrontation* (vs. interpretation) as necessarily the most effective means to achieve it (e.g., the discussion of response to the first crisis with Ali over looking at her legs, and the conclusions); and (2) the related implication that deliberate, manifest *assertions of the analyst's subjectivity*—as it differs from that of the patient (albeit, selectively, Holly makes clear)—is quite as universally a part of the enacted communications that convey the analyst's "compassion," and even the patient's "impact" on the analyst.

Let me be totally clear. The elements of analytic communication—affective honesty, compassion, impact on the analyst—that Holly privileges are, as I see it, absolutely central and vital. These qualities constitute much of the universal, deep relational structure of a useful analysis—beyond, in my view, manifest differences in style and technique. Holly's responses to Ali stylistically resemble the work of analysts like Bromberg, Davies, Ehrenberg, Hoffman, and Renik, and, in my view, seem to convey these universal human values as fully and effectively as we see (unfortunately, not commonly) in analytic work. Yet, if we read Holly as implying that various *other* ways of conceptualizing the intersubjective clash with Ali and responding to it would—for *other* analysts—necessarily be experienced as "absenting" themselves from the experience with Ali in ways that "would have lost her", I am not sure that, as a general principle, I would fully agree.

Holly believes that any analyst working with Ali without engaging in Holly's particular kind of expressive confrontation might "lose her." So it might be useful to look at the story of Ali and Holly to envision other ways of making and sustaining an analytic relationship that may be usefully practiced by different analysts in different "analytic couples." Is there a certain range of therapeutically fruitful—yet still profoundly "affectively honest"—styles of response that are less confrontative than Holly's and the tradition she shares? Are these other relational styles embedded in slightly different views of intersubjectivity?

Holly says that she is drawing on multiple meanings of intersubjectivity, though primarily those of Benjamin. As I see it, Holly's basic assumptions seem fundamentally compatible with Benjamin's (1990) developmental version of "intersubjectivity" in which there is a universal need to transcend the dynamic of domination/subjugation that is assumed to be intrinsic to the problem of Otherness. In contrast, Holly's intersubjective sensibility shares less with the self psychological version of intersubjectivity of Stolorow, Brandchaft, and Atwood (1987), in which manifest, intersubjective clashes (and the types of enactments they may entail) are seen as rooted in differing subjective worlds, frames of meaning, and types of self-organization. There is no assumption here that intersubjective clashes are derivative of a presumed universal, relational power dynamic. I'll try briefly to spell out these issues by imagining some of the ways other analysts who envision intersubjectivity differently might conceivably have responded to Ali.

Holly's Legs: Responding to What Appears to be an Envious (Coercive) Effort to "Take" From the Analyst

Starting with her depiction of her encounter with Ali on the staircase and her own complex inner process following it, Holly's work seems to me to be an excellent example of one way in which a resourceful, creative analyst makes use of destabilizing clashes between her subjectivity and that of her patient. She widens her access to her own inner experience and becomes aware of an important interactive dynamic between them. The process flows like this:

Holly feels misunderstood about Ali's implication that Holly wants to exhibit her legs, yet is unable to perform what will inevitably seem like a defensive denial, or, as she feels it, an evasion (perhaps cast in the form of an "interpretation") of such desire. After considerable inner struggle to become more fully aware of the range of her own feelings, Holly responds to Ali in a way that communicates both her sense of Ali's larger experience of deprivation, *and* Holly's view that Ali believes she will "never get anything unless [she] takes it." Holly then explains that for her personally as well as, it is implied, for most people, being approached in this grabby, peremptory way will be unlikely to produce the giving response that Ali desires; rather, it will provoke from Holly and, potentially, most others in Ali's life, a reactive urge to withhold.

This communication seems to touch Ali deeply. She cries, initially feels abandoned, seems reassured by Holly's heartfelt disclaimer of any intent to reject her, and finally tells Holly how meaningful the episode was. Her response also seems to be profoundly centering for Holly. It has allowed her to show Ali something of the live, immediate, internal struggle in which Holly is engaged: that is, sensing Ali's pain and caring for her, yet feeling cut off by Ali's aggressive demands from her own acknowledged inner desire to give freely.

As I see it, this interaction—viewed in the context of their relationship and of Holly's inner experience—is a beautiful example of what Holly advocates as "affective honesty" and compassionate communication. Although she doesn't spell it out, I think Holly implies (and my own experience corroborates) that in experiencing her complex impact on the analyst in this emotional context, Ali is also moved to reflect more clearly and usefully on herself.

The Meaning of Enactment Around Envy, Hate, and Love Through a Nonrelational Lens

As I read and savor Holly's bold and thoughtful confrontation, I nevertheless find myself imagining productive interactions between Ali and other hypothetical analysts unfolding in a variety of ways. Some might *sound like* the confrontation around envy and coercion but actually mean something very different to Ali. Others might sound manifestly different from Holly's words and yet convey much of what I see as some of the most critical and universally applicable aspects of Holly's approach: its hard-won affective honesty, compassion, and expressive depiction of the patient's impact on the analyst.

It's easy to imagine many less relational analysts responding to Ali's comments about their legs (or the equivalent) in a fashion that initially sounds as if it were conveying some of the same content but deriving from a totally different analytic paradigm. For example, the Kleinians often focus on patients' communications that strike the analyst as intending to "coerce," a personally expressive response. Typically viewed as "projective identifications," the assumption is that such communications are often rooted in paranoid beliefs about the analyst's intentions and the patient's envious wishes to undermine analytic authority and the analytic process (Bott-Spillius, 1988; Joseph, 1989). I can envision such analysts conveying something that might even sound similar to Holly's confrontative "I wonder if you believe you'll never get anything unless you take it ... envy doesn't work that way."

To be sure, my imagined Kleinian analyst will virtually never follow up the confrontation with a heartfelt assurance like Holly's "I will give it to you if I want to—you just have to let me do it in my own time." While Holly seems to believe she can, in fact, provide some of the love Ali desires, Kleinian views of the dynamics of envy and coercive projective identification would probably interpret Holly's promise to give "in my own time" as failing to identify Ali's entrapment in core, pathological convictions about the destructiveness of her own desires and the belief that the analyst must want to deprive and punish her for them. Encouraging the patient to believe that by modifying her overt behavior—her demandingness—she can fit the analyst's preconditions for giving love, might be seen as reinforcing Ali's belief that, in fact, the analyst does hate her (at least the greedy part of her) and cannot tolerate her rage. In Kleinian terms, the enactment might be seen as an unwitting repetition of a coercive, parental, developmental interaction. In this scenario, Ali remains stuck with a split, paranoid vision of the analyst as either a teasing, depriving Other, or an omnipotent provider of an illusory forgiveness and acceptance. Fully experiencing the world—the breast—as a giving as well as a depriving object and experiencing oneself as genuinely worthy of love cannot come from Holly's candid expression of the conditionality of her love. It can only emerge from the patient's inner confrontation with her own fantasized destructiveness.

To address the destructive side of envy, Kleinian theory both minimizes the power of the analyst's emotional response as an important new, transformative, human reality and at the same time privileges the analyst's theoretical/technical frame as an objective representation of the patient's inner truth. Holly, on the other hand, is not constrained by a theoretical context that defines the intersubjective analytic relationship (and the powerful, mutual feelings of love and hate in it) as somehow *less real*—or less therapeutically significant—than a presumed set of unconscious fantasies within Ali's mind. In addressing what she, like the Kleinians, sees as the central destructiveness/self-destructiveness in Ali's demanding envy, Holly is less concerned with the possibility that she is engaged in a new form of coercion, a new form of unwitting "pathological enactment." Holly does not conceive of their enactment as a repetition of something omnipotent and old but, rather, as the analyst's creative use of her own emotional responsiveness as the vehicle by which both participants will initially move on to negotiate new meanings.

Perhaps we could narrate Holly's version of the enactment as follows: Initially, Holly suffered Ali's aggressive characterization of her needing to draw Ali's gaze to her legs as a violation of Holly's subjective sense of her own motives as well as a demand for her love. Holly then struggled to find a way for her own subjectivity to "survive" what she experienced as Ali's misconstruals of her identity by recognizing something more basic in her experience: the conflict over giving and withdrawing that Holly feels stirred in her, and the way this conflict seems to provoke a painful inhibition of her own positive responsiveness. Holly then created her own vehicle for expressing her psychological survival in the form of a confrontation that communicates both her love and her hate for Ali as well as her view of their conflict is a clash of interpersonal strategies for negotiating affective responses. Holly then communicates from her "recentered" vantage point with a new offer: greater responsiveness from Holly (and, potentially, the world at large) in exchange for a shift by Ali towards a less aggressive negotiating strategy.

Holly's ultimate response to Ali emerged from a complex, inner process of internal and interpersonal conflict, a loss of stability and clarity, and, eventually, a recentering around issues in the analytic relationship that had initially destabilized and deeply confused her. I think Holly's capacity to suffer through a period of personal exploration to arrive at a way of understanding and communicating creatively with Ali is at the heart of what is effective in her work. I think, too, that her capacity to arrive at her exceptional affective honesty is somewhat separable from (a) Holly's particular strategy for finding the Other as well as (b) her distinctive form of expressing her Otherness through candid confrontation and negotiated giving. To make clearer what I mean by suggesting that the key elements of what we see in Holly's process are somewhat separable from the particular content and style of Holly's response, consider how still another analyst might respond in a manifestly very different way to Ali's comments about her wanting her to see Holly's legs.

Affective Honesty, Confrontation, and Interpretation in an Alternative Intersubjective Context

Imagine this time an analyst who, like Holly, feels that her subjectivity is misread by Ali and who senses, as well, the aggressive quality in Ali's effort to coerce her into admitting to seductive intent by showing her legs. Suppose this analyst finds herself initially angry, confused, and inhibited. Then, in contrast to Holly's move towards understanding their intersubjective conflict as rooted in Ali's counterproductive negotiating strategy, this other analyst moves into her initial turmoil, perhaps her own deepened "depressive anxiety," in a way that wrenches her away from her own subjective center—away even from the intensity with which she bridles at Ali's characterization of her erotic narcissism. In the course of this, "analyst X," we'll call her, realizes that there may be fundamental and radical differences in how she and Ali have been organizing the whole experience of their struggle.

A different set of meanings emerge: What is being "enacted" between Ali and analyst X is seen as actually initiated by a striving on Ali's part to communicate an elemental need to establish and affirm the realness, aliveness, and nonexploitativeness of the connection between them. Ali's "desire to be the object of Holly's desire" (a need that Holly identifies but does not stress) is seen by analyst X as an attempt to find the erotic response that Ali sorely missed with her father but to find it through a feisty self-assertion rather than by becoming the overprotective caretaker of the other—the price mother had imposed for her love. Analyst X slowly realizes that, in her mother's aggressive demand for merger, it was Ali who felt coerced to have the feelings mother needed from her, quite like analyst X felt coerced to have and acknowledge exactly the feelings that Ali needed her to have.

"Look, Ali," says this hypothetical analyst, "maybe you're actually sensing something in me when you say I *wanted* you to look at my legs, something that goes beyond what I'm aware of. But, as I think about it, it feels to me that maybe what you're getting at is how much you want to feel that what I feel for you is real and that I really welcome your passion in seeing me and your feeling for me. My desire would be something powerful that draws me to you in a way that you could never feel from your father. That visceral attraction sometimes feels like *the* thing, the only thing that you can trust will *hold* me or anyone in a way that can be relied on, over time, no matter what." And somewhere, some time in all this the analyst adds, "when you challenge me in your feisty way to admit it, you don't have to worry about playing once again the good girl who needs to take care of mom." At some point, later—perhaps in the third crisis that Holly describes as revolving around their separations—analyst X adds that, "Sometimes it seems like you feel that the only way we can bear the pain of our separations and stay connected through them is if—as your mother required—the emotions we feel are identical."

For analyst X, attributing these new meanings serves to recognize not only Ali's subjective world but, significantly, to reframe the analyst's self experience as well. The analyst has understood their differences, their intersubjective clash, in a way that first of all alleviates her sense that her own awareness of her desires needs to be complete and without self-deception. Beyond that, she feels much less the need to *provide* Ali with responses that, like Holly, analyst X knows that she cannot provide. In her way, she's trying to survive the challenge to her subjectivity through decentering temporarily from it. She does not leave her subjectivity but rather finds in herself—through the act of decentering—a version of the patient's subjectivity (and a reciprocal version of her own) that, in a different way from Holly, she too brings to the negotiating table as an "offer" for Ali.

I hope it is amply clear that I do not offer this alternative as a better response but merely to illustrate how a different intersubjective process might, in its own way, convey the analyst's compassionate struggle and express the patient's impact on her. Apart from what we may judge to be its correctness, or its complex connection to Ali's history, many of us would think of analyst X's response as more "interpretive" than enactive. At least some aspects of her approach are interpretations rooted in analyst X's emotional acceptance of Ali's otherness and her recognition of her patient's distinct, subjective frame of meaning.

Would analyst X be communicating with affective honesty? She might be—since I've imagined her, like Holly, able to let the power of the intersubjective process jostle her loose from her own subjective world and, with her theory as a rough guide, able to recreate her new subjective vantage point. But only, I think, if we imagine analyst X venturing her interpretations in the spirit of showing the patient her (the analyst's) own mind at work—showing the patient, as Winnicott (1950) put it ironically, the limits of the analyst's own understanding.

Still More Meanings of Enactment and Interpretation

Is analyst X enacting something? Some might say that she is, in effect, communicating through a powerful enactment but an enactment in a very different sense from Holly's. Enactment here might be seen as the *needed enactment* of a developmental scenario in which Ali experiences the recognition of something that has always pervaded her quest for an erotic response as well as for an Other who does not need her subjectivity either to coincide with or to clash with, Ali's. Therapeutic enactment in this alternative view of intersubjectivity—one that is closer to Stolorow and Atwood's (1987) than it is to Benjamin's (1990)—is in a sense still central. Rightly or wrongly, this view differs from what I believe is, by and large, the message of Holly's narrative: that it is in the confrontation of the inevitable clash of subjectivities that we find the therapeutically more useful conflictual enactments.

Neither the interpretative elements of analyst X's response nor the form of enactment of the needed relationship are derived from the classical wish/defense paradigm, nor do they confront directly the conflicting aspects of the subjectivities of analyst and patient. Rather, the interpretations delineate what are possibly deeper strivings that have been regularly frustrated—strivings for a reliable affective signal, an erotic signal, from the object as well as strivings for a freedom from coercion into mirrored or merged emotions with the Other. All of these strivings may, in a sense, be relatively accessible to Ali's experience but so regularly dressed in her feisty and peremptory demands that they are easily missed by others, as well as by Ali herself.

Ironically, if some "interpretive" understandings such as these are simultaneously personally expressive, so too what is so personally expressive in Holly's more obviously confrontative enactment also becomes "interpretative" in that it, too, is an effort to understand Ali's behavior in light of a larger framework of meaning. In the first of the three intersubjective clashes with Ali that are discussed, Holly conveys to Ali a view of how the interpersonal world universally works much better when we don't try to control it; and, more specifically, how Ali's violation of this norm reduces her chances of getting the world to respond as she wishes. In the third critical moment, the theme of mortality is introduced by Ali's fears for Holly's health and links up in multiple ways with Holly's personal experiences of loss. What Holly conveys to Ali—though rooted in references to the enacted experience of their relationship—is, again, quite interpretive. Holly confronts the real conflicts between their subjectivities—in this case Ali's implicit expectation that they must be merged in their reactions to separation in order to bear its pain. Yet Holly couples this with a broad, interpretive understanding of how Ali has never been helped by her parents to learn to deal with the inevitable elements of separation and loss as aspects of all attachments.

Observing the interpretive elements in Holly's form of personal expressiveness and the potential for personal expressiveness—affective honesty as well as affective hiding—in different interpretive communications, nudges me toward a view that emphasizes the meaning of the underlying intersubjective message, rather than the manifest form (whether interpretation, confrontation, or enactment) in which the message is delivered. Because the manifest form of the message (i.e., interpretation) is privileged in more traditional analytic views (views that often seem oblivious to inherent performative, enactive meanings), it seems to me that we need to be careful not to compound the problem by valorizing "noninterpretive" vehicles of communication as somehow radically different from interpretive and cognitive messages. In emphasizing interactive (procedural, implicit) communication, we can miss the often profoundly interpretive elements within enactments that take an outwardly personal, expressive form.

Affective Honesty, Impact on the Analyst, and Compassion

As I see it, the core problem that Holly addresses throughout her article is how analysts can best make use of (make into usable self knowledge for their patients) the intersubjective clashes that analysts experience in the analytic relationship, especially those clashes that seem most directly to challenge aspects (sometimes dissociated aspects) of the analyst's own identity. More specifically, Holly addresses how this can be done in a way that the patient experiences as having an impact on the analyst and as affectively honest and compassionate. If I look at my own work and extend that work with data from the (sometimes strikingly) different, yet often strikingly successful, work of my long-term supervisees, I continually see patients like Ali asking us to try to go somewhere—emotionally, imaginatively, ethically—beyond where, in virtually any other human relationship, we are ready to go. The analytic frame, theory, and technique certainly serve us and protect us—to a degree—but in a way that I think actually also puts us in greater emotional jeopardy. Sometimes we must simply tolerate and suffer more—or quite differently—than we do in any other of life's relational contexts.

Whether this comes in the form of a set of crunch-like crises like those of Holly and Ali or simply in the form of subtle, long-term shifts in the building of a relationship, my sense is that analysts are usually called on to revisit their own basic versions of certain core, human existential issues. I am not talking about the analyst's issues in the sense of fixed countertransference problems within the analyst's psyche. Rather, I am referring to a more intersubjective phenomenon: to relate deeply to a given patient, like Ali, many tensions within the analyst may have to be reopened, despite the fact that the analyst may well have resolved those tensions quite sufficiently to function well in the rest of the analyst's life. In one form or another we end up feeling compelled to produce, or share, or bear some view of ourselves—some response—that the patient seems desperately to need.

Ali needs to feel she is desired in a particular way by Holly; she rages at her own idealized view of Holly's life and calls for Holly to experience their identities as merged in the mortal dread of not surviving their separation. But, to maintain her hold on her separate reality (her Otherness)—indeed to extract what in these moments her Otherness she may actually offer to her patient—Holly knows that there is something about Ali's reality, about at least the form in which Ali's needs are expressed, that she *cannot* accept. In its present form, there is something she feels she must *refuse*.

If Holly doesn't find a visible, expressible way to join Ali's reality, there is a sense in which she may abandon her. Yet, it *seems* that to join her Holly must violate her own needs, indeed sometimes whole tracts of her subjective reality and her privacy. Often it can seem as though joining her implies violating the analytic role and the frame itself.

Most analysts will, like Holly, sometimes experience such intersubjective clashes as tormenting, mind-bending, emotional double binds. Theories and favored technical styles—whether they are manifestly confrontative, interpretive, or empathic—are desperately needed at these times to hold and contain analyst and patient while they try to work on the conflict and paradox that pervades these experiences. Yet, while legitimating and sustaining us through these challenges, our theories ultimately can't obscure the fact that those very interactions that may feel coercive may well entail the vital human need to see who *we* are and what kind of potentially "new" experience our patients can have with us (Aron, 1996; Slavin and Kriegman,1998).

Patients like Ali can be seen as using a wide range of human interactive capacities (learned relational tactics, projections, role inductions) as ways of compelling us as analysts to experience *ourselves* more fully and, if we are capable, to confront and struggle with real tensions within ourselves. Analysts may reciprocate by opening the *analyst's own versions* of the same human dilemmas (around what is real, love and hate, risk and attachment, mortality, despair) that prove overwhelming for the patient and are, for all of us, ongoing, lifelong human adaptive challenges with which we never cease to grapple (Slavin, 2003, 2005).

Therapeutic Action and the Enactment of Developmental Conflicts

As I see it, this kind of intersubjective negotiation is closely akin to what goes on around key developmental challenges and transitions between parents and children. We know that parents inevitably struggle with (and often defend against struggling with) the reopening of their own inner working solutions to the very issues currently facing their children. The personal realness of this mutual challenge for the analyst and patient is what replicates the intersubjective context—the interactive conditions in the family—in which the patient's less adaptive solutions were shaped.

I think we *become* usable transferential versions of parents when in some measure we have, like Holly (or, in a very different manifest style, like my imagined analyst X), allowed ourselves to become a bit lost in our versions of precisely those developmental challenges where our patients' earlier experiences with parental figures in the family failed them. Throughout the crises in this analysis—around whether Holly needed Ali to desire and admire her, around the tensions over Ali's envious idealizations, and around the mortal anxiety over their separations—Ali seemed enabled to revisit and perhaps revise old conclusions about love and identity through a relational process that entailed the analyst's willingness to reopen, revisit, and *suffer anew* something *old* in herself. In the context of this reliving, Holly seemed to rediscover her own genuine, personal conditions for feeling (and not feeling) love, as well as re-recognize the mixture of hate and poignant loss that love inevitably entails. What seemed key was Holly's signaling her willingness to create a more level playing field—a field of two fellow sufferers, each dealing with their own limits, sadness, and hope, bringing to bear their differing strengths and roles to grapple reciprocally with the same human dilemmas. I think of what they did as a type of mutually induced opening up and experiencing of the patient's own struggles in the altered context of a strong and competent Other—an Other who is, nevertheless, able to allow herself to be similarly engaged and open to developmental change.

Analysts may discover their own inner sense of limits, sadness, and hope (a deepened experience by the analyst of depressive anxiety) in different ways. Some, like Holly, will achieve this affective honesty in a way that finds its integrity in expressing itself through selective self-disclosure and confrontation (and, I think, *implicit* interpretation) of what the analyst views as a coercive, driven, false intimacy, and merged mirroring. Other analysts—like my imagined, hypothetical analyst X—will emerge from this deepened depressive anxiety, if you will, through a radical re-experiencing of the patient's needs and a reframed definition of the patient's subjective strivings that, itself, conveys the deep impact the patient has had on the analyst. The meanings of intersubjective conflict between analyst and patient are re-envisioned in terms of the patient's underlying developmental strivings and are, in a sense, *manifested* as interpretations.

I clearly sense that Holly (and I would hope my imagined analyst X) emerged from this treatment with a clearer sense of her own perceptions, the validity of her own needs, and a deeper appreciation of both her own agency and mortality. She has arrived here by courageously allowing some of Ali's vigorous intersubjective probes to destabilize her and by wholeheartedly engaging in a mutual process of renegotiating aspects of herself to help Ali find the sources of her own growth.

Although we sometimes speak of a kind of healing of the analyst that goes on when we engage in this way, I think Searles (1975) classic discussion of the patient as "therapist to the therapist" construed this process far too narrowly. While the impact on the analyst may be seen as constituting a therapeutic act, it is perhaps better understood as encompassing an important source of potential adult developmental growth (Levinson, 1976) that may come from a deep, personal engagement in our work. It is this growth, this process of risk and change, and impact out of which Holly's creative work with Ali has crystallized that generates the particular form of affective honesty and compassion we see shining from Holly's work.

REFERENCES

Aron, L. (1996), *A Meeting of Minds: Mutuality in Psychoanalysis*. Hillsdale, NJ: The Analytic Press.

Benjamin, J. (1990), Recognition and destruction: An outline of intersubjectivity. In: *Relational Perspectives in Psychoanalysis*, eds. N. J. Skolnick & S. C. Warshaw, Hillsdale, NJ: The Analytic Press, pp. 43–60.

Bott-Spillius, E. (1988), *Melanie Klein Today: Developments in Theory and Practice*. London: Routledge.

Joseph, B. (1989), *Psychic Equilibrium and Psychic Change*. London: Tavistock/Rouledge.

Levinson, D. (1976), *The Seasons of a Man's Life*. New York: Ballantine.

Russell, P. Crises of emotional growth [a.k.a. the theory of the crunch] (unpublished manuscript).

Searles, H. F. (1975), The patient as therapist to his analyst. In: *Tactics and Techniques in Psychoanalytic Theory. Volume II: Countertransference*, ed. P. Giovacchini. New York: Aronson, pp. 95–151.

Slavin, M. (2003), How We Struggle To Become "New Objects". Discussion of Jody Messler Davies' "Whose Bad Objects Are These Anyway? Repetition and Our Elusive Love Affair with Evil." IARPP Conference, Toronto, Canada, January, 2003.

_____ (2005), Afterword to Chapter, "Why the analyst needs to change; toward a theory of conflict, negotiation and mutual influence in the therapeutic relationship." In: *Relational Psychoanalysis II*, eds. L. Aron. & A. Harris. Hillsdale, NJ: The Analytic Press, pp. 75–119.

_____ & Kriegman, D. (1998), Why the analyst needs to change; toward a theory of conflict, negotiation and mutual influence in the therapeutic relationship. *Psychoanalytic Dialogues*, 8:247–284.

Stolorow, R., Brandchaft, B., & Atwood, G. (1987), *Psychoanalytic Treatment: An Intersubjective Approach*. Hillsdale, NJ: The Analytic Press.

Winnicott, D. W. (1950), *Hate in the countertransference. Through Paediatrics to Psychoanalysis*. New York: Basic Books. 1975.

112 Lakeview Avenue
Cambridge, MA 02138
malslavin@aol.com

"Affective Honesty" as Example and Metaphor: Discussion of Holly Levenkron's "Love (and Hate) With the Proper Stranger: Affective Honesty and Enactment"

DONNEL B. STERN, PH.D.

Levenkron begins with the thesis that the analyst is never outside of enactments between herself and her patient. The analyst must enage these enactments with affective honesty, and this must be done during the sessions within which the events in question occur (i.e., in the heat of the moment, without necessarily being able to formulate the relevant unconscious meanings). Levenkron's contribution is her recognition of the necessity for the confrontation created by the analyst's affectively honest reaction to the attempt by both the patient and herself to force the relationship along certain paths.

Donnel B. Stern, Ph.D. is Editor of *Contemporary Psychoanalysis;* Editor of "Psychoanalysis in a New Key" Book Series (The Analytic Press); Training and Supervising Analyst at the William Alanson White Institute, New York City; and Faculty member of the New York University Postdoctoral Program in Psychotherapy and Psychoanalysis. He is the author of *Unformulated Experience: From Dissociation to Imagination in Psychoanalysis* (The Analytic Press, 1997) and co-editor of *The Handbook of Interpersonal Psychoanalysis* (The Analytic Press, 1995). He serves on the editorial boards of *Psychoanalytic Inquiry, Psychoanalytic Dialogues,* and *Psychoanalytic Psychology.*

IN HER FINELY TEXTURED AND NUANCED ACCOUNT OF SESSIONS WITH her patient Ali, Holly Levenkron is unusually successful in finding words for her own subtle feelings and perceptions, and she conveys her grasp of Ali's with equal specificity and delicacy. When Levenkron describes an interaction, we can actually feel what is happening from moment to moment. I admire this article for these novelistic qualities alone. But there is more here than compelling prose. Levenkron uses her experience-near account of her clinical experience to present a perspective on clinical work—an interesting and useful perspective, even an inspiring one. And she doesn't just present the perspective. She lays out her experience with Ali in such a way that we can see exactly how she came to her views.

This is rare. Seldom do we have the opportunity to follow along with a thoughtful, creative, and seasoned clinician as she formulates her ideas about how she works and why she feels that her approach is a useful way to go about it. More often what we read are the ideas that authors distill from raw experiences, ideas that, by the time they are worked out on the page, are far removed from the circumstances that provoked them. Why? First, because writing in the way Levenkron has written has not been acceptable in psychoanalysis until recently. As long as psychoanalysis needed to be science and we were ashamed to be caught acting on something other than (what we believed was) a defensible theory of technique, the inevitably personal roots of theory had to be camouflaged. That is how we ended up, for example, with Kohut's (1979) curious "The Two Analyses of Mr. Z," in which, as we discovered many years after the article was published, Mr. Z. turns out to be Kohut himself. Given the state of American psychoanalysis in his day (and that was not very long ago), Kohut couldn't justify the risk of talking about his own experience of narcissism and how convincing it was. It would be painfully difficult to do that even today.

Though the general reluctance to acknowledge the personal in our work has diminished since the 1970s, frankness can still be dangerous to your health. Writing as Levenkron has written here is risky. People are not always rewarded for honesty, and this article required an unusual degree of it. Levenkron reveals personal matters that most of us keep to ourselves, and she does it without wafting our way even a whiff of sensationalism or exhibitionism. We profit from her revelations; they contribute to her theme.

One of the reasons none of her revelations seems gratuitous or self-aggrandizing is that Levenkron seems to have no agenda in her article other than to tell us what she did and why she did it. Despite the fact that her article is positioned at the leading edge of the relational changes going on in American psychoanalysis today, there is no proselytizing here, no band-wagon brouhaha. Levenkron simply tells us how she thought and felt her way into the kind of work she did. She is as honest with us as she is with Ali, and we receive her article with the same recognition of its authenticity as Ali seems to have felt about Levenkron in some of the clinical episodes. As I think is often the case with good clinical writing, the article itself is an instance of the kind of work described in it. Levenkron adopts no ironclad rules about how much or how little to tell either Ali or us, and then she does what she believes is best for the treatment (or the article) in each instance, accompanying what she does with enough of its context that we, and Ali too, can see why she chooses to do it.

The substance of Levenkron's view is straightforward: since the analyst is never outside enactments, she cannot wait until an enactment ends to deal with it (as Levenkron agrees, enactments never end really; they just change, so that the point where you choose to say that one has ceased and the next has begun is arbitrary). She must do whatever she is going to do from within the enactment, as it takes place, and she does that by finding her way to the "affective honesty" that is necessary to negotiate between her own desires and those of the analysand's. Desire is the mainspring of enactments and the reason they are continuous and inevitable. Each person continuously exerts conscious and unconscious influence on the other to recognize and satisfy her desire. The choreography of engaged desires is enactment.

The influences on this view are clear enough (and Levenkron cites them); but exactly where the influences end and Levenkron's own view begins would be hard to establish—if one cared to try, which I don't. Woven throughout we see, among other important ideas, Benjamin's (e.g., 1990, 1999) thinking on intersubjectivity; Ehrenberg's (1992) style of working on "the intimate edge" and her focus on desire in the interpersonal field; Bromberg's (1998) understanding of the centrality of engagement and en-actment; Bromberg's (1998) and Pizer's (1998) work on the negotiation of enactments (joined now by my own work on the subject—Stern, 2003, 2004); the focus by Slavin and Kriegman (1998) on conflict and negotia-tion as the heart of clinical relatedness; and Renik's (1993, 1995) insistence on the inevitability of the personal and subjective. In the end, though, Levenkron's particular distillation of these resources is her own. The spe-cial kind of confrontation opened up by what she calls "affective honesty" is Levenkron's contribution to our understanding of what it takes to shift the struggles for domination that make up enactments into something different, something more like two people each recognizing the other's separate subjectivity (Benjamin, 1990), even if neither likes what they see.

It isn't accidental that I cite the work of others in describing Levenkron's argument. I have the impression that Levenkron didn't set out to contribute an original theoretical perspective but to offer an illustration of how the relational principles she admires in the contributions of others might work in practice—her own, very personal kind of practice. The value of the article lies in its example: it is a way of working for us to consult, in our minds, as we sit with our patients, as we try to work out our own ways of conducting psychoanalytic work. "Affective honesty" is one of those many metaphors we access at those times, hoping that one of them will help us see and feel what we cannot yet see and feel.

It has been clear to relational and interpersonal analysts for a number of years now that, in each moment, we have no choice but to select one of the personal responses available to us (though of course those personal responses include interventions of the traditional kind); there is no objective "platform" (Mitchell, 1997) or "perch" (Modell, 1991) upon which it is possible for the analyst to retreat from subjectivity. The process of selecting which of these personal responses to employ is understood by most of these analysts to be a search for the analyst's authentic responsiveness to the patient; and in this sense authenticity has assumed the place that technical correctness once held. But which authenticity? There are any number of authentic responses Levenkron could have made to Ali in these vignettes, and by no means would all of them have been useful. How should the analyst make her selection?

Levenkron's article, thankfully, is not an attempt to answer this question, which is unanswerable outside a specific clinical context. (More accurately, it is *unaddressable* outside a specific clinical context, since even when the context is specified the answer often remains elusive.) Levenkron tells us about affective honesty in a way that allows us to recognize it in her examples, but she neither encourages us to theorize about it, nor to believe we can generate it at will. Affective honesty is not an algorithm for selecting a clinical response. The idea will help those clinicians with whom it resonates, as it does for me; but the particular shape of affective honesty, and the moments of its appearance, must always be unforeseeable. The analyst never knows when she will suddenly find herself able to destabilize an enactment, and often enough she finds out only in retrospect that she has done so. Even authenticity, that is, is a contextual matter (Mitchell, 1993, 123–150).

The measure of an article is whether it makes you think differently about your work. Several times since I read Levenkron's article, as I have been sitting with a patient and feeling the grip of the field tightening on us uncomfortably, I have asked myself something like, "Now, what is it that he wants from me, and that maybe I don't want to give him; and what do I want from him that maybe he doesn't want to give me? How might I put these things into words in a way that would respect his wishes while at the same time continuing to respect my own?"

In one of these instances, I was trying to reschedule an appointment with a patient, an appointment I had been the one to cancel. My patient, Doris, was a highly intelligent middle-aged professional woman whom I had seen for quite some time and with whom there had been frequent and bitter conflict over what she felt was my overvaluation of my own views and wishes and my disregard, dismissal, and misinterpretation of hers. At the same time, Doris was someone I respected and with whom I often felt quite close, and I know she feels these same things about me. I am aware of how much she values the treatment, and that awareness includes knowing how difficult it is for her to pay for each session. I have special reasons, that is, to want to offer Doris make-up appointments.

I offered Doris several alternative meeting times on this occasion, apparently more than she expected. Angrily and accusingly, she told me that when she had cancelled a session I had never made such accommodations, offered so many alternative times. She suggested that I was willing to try harder to satisfy my own desire for income than to satisfy her desire for a make-up session. That certainly seemed possible to me, but I also knew, as I have said, that I had often gone to greater lengths to reschedule her missed appointments than I had with other patients, sometimes giving her make-up times several weeks away from the session she missed (which I don't do otherwise, an enactment in itself). On those occasions when I had not made up a missed session, I had told her that I did not have the time to give her. I felt now that she was also implying that I had been lying, that the availability of my time *now* indicated to her that I had the time *then*. I just wouldn't give it to her.

I told Doris that I could see why the fact that I had more hours to offer her now required some kind of explanation and asked her whether it had occurred to her that there might be any other reason than the one she seemed to be considering. Fuming, she indicated that she thought she knew what the explanation was: in the past, when I had not made up appointments, I had seen an opportunity to use her sessions for other activities, like writing, and be paid for them anyway. It wouldn't have served my purposes to give her a make-up.

With a certain degree of heat I replied that, in that case, considering that I had told her quite explicitly that I had no time to offer her, I had to conclude that she was accusing me of having lied to her. She said she wasn't accusing me of anything and that now *I* seemed angry at *her* (which was right). That wasn't fair, she said. *She* was the one who had the right to be angry at *me*! Wasn't she supposed to say what she was thinking? What should she do, just keep something to herself if she thought it might bother me?

I was not feeling my calmest or most articulate. I had Levenkron's article in recent memory, though. I asked myself what it was that my patient wanted from me. In the immediate sense, at least, it seemed to me that she wanted me to say that she was right and I was wrong, that I refused to recognize the validity of her position, that in the service of my own wishes I was willing to disregard her desires so thoroughly that I would lie to do it. (It was her observation, later on, that this is exactly what she believes about her father.)

And what did I want from her? I felt mistreated, just as she did. I wanted her to acknowledge that, in fact, I was a pretty good guy, certainly honest with someone I knew as well and cared about as much as her. Maybe I even wanted her to give me credit for a certain degree of generosity, for going out of my way for her—though she didn't know about that then. I wanted her to see me as I saw myself. In other words, I wanted *her* to recognize *me*, to admit that *I* was right.

I didn't describe these thoughts to Doris in so many words. Levenkron's way of thinking was one of the things that allowed me to step back and create a space to think in, and it helped me to bring myself back to the clinical task. The symmetry in our attempt to dominate one another, what Benjamin would call "complementarity," gave me pause and helped me to recognize that something different had to happen. When I did speak, I was able to do so with some of the equanimity I had lost. I had at least partially breached the dissociation that cordoned off the enactment from the rest of my experience of the relatedness between Doris and me. (In many respects, Levenkron's conception of enactment as dissociation mirrors my own [Stern, 2003, 2004]). What I said, which was more or less the following, was rooted in the thoughts Levenkron's article had stimulated in me:

You say you're not accusing me of lying. But let's be straightforward. You're suspicious of me. You've always been suspicious of me. You worry that you can't trust me to tell you the truth about my self-interest and how it affects what I'm willing to give you. You worry that I don't even *know* the truth, that I don't grasp the extent of my own narcissism. You suggest that I've lied to you, and then you feel it's unfair of me to react to what you say, as if my reacting to it means that I think you shouldn't have said it. Of course you should say it, if it's what you're thinking. But you can't expect to tell a person who wants to think of himself as honest—and that's me—that he's a liar without arousing a reaction. It's a pretty serious accusation. You feel I'm lying, and I react with anger. You want me to say you're right, and I want you to say you're wrong.

But we don't have to be bound by that; that's only the way it started. Let's see what we can do with it. Let's just talk about it straightforwardly, accepting that it's not pleasant and that probably both of us would rather feel otherwise.

A number of things came of this intervention, which, while not as pithy as the things Levenkron said to Ali, seems to me to echo it, especially my willingness to confront Doris with the fact that both her experience and mine were significant and that we both needed to pay attention to what was going on with both of us. (She would say, incidentally, that I, too, hadn't been willing to pay attention to what was going on with both of us, and she'd be as right as I'd been.)

When Doris repeated that she couldn't imagine an alternative explanation for the sudden availability of make-up times, I asked her if it was really so inconceivable to her that I would have some empty hours once in a while. Well, she said, in fact she *had* thought of that, but she'd kept it to herself. She hadn't even really made it into a thought. Why? Because she thought *that* would *really* bother me, and she wanted to avoid either hurting me or making me angry!

I was dumbstruck. How narcissistic could she imagine me to be? Apparently she believed that I would feel worse about revealing that I had unfilled hours than I would about being accused of lying!

As you might imagine, all of this expanded in more directions than I can develop here. Doris's parents, each for a different reason and in different ways, had treated her during childhood as if her wishes and needs were burdensome and exploitative, so that now she tends to deny self-interest, often sacrificing her own desires before she even lets herself know she has them. When she does experience self-interest, she is liable to feel wrong, or even disgusting; and with the same consistency, the other's self-interest is depriving, hurtful, and enraging. On a deeper level of the enactment around the make-up—a level of issues that Doris and I eventually found our way to discussing—Doris wanted me to care for her enough and to have enough empathic connection with the depth of her need to make whatever accommodations were necessary to give her what she wanted so badly—in this case, make-up sessions. She wanted her wishes to be at least as important to me as my own. No, *more* important. She wanted me to care about her wishes in a way that she can't do herself.

That is something I couldn't and can't do; but I can now see my way more easily to staying in touch with the depth of her need. I have less difficulty acknowledging to myself that my interests sometimes hurt her simply by existing, at least when they conflict with hers. I am more able to know, even when Doris is not acting that way, that she is *afflicted* by her own desire, as if it were some kind of shameful disease.

No matter how useful any way of looking at enactments is, however, in the end we have the same problem: how do we get to the state in which we are able to offer a negotiation that has a reasonable chance of destabilizing the ossified relatedness? While we can agree that the state in which affective honesty becomes possible is a good thing, we still must find our way to that state; and in the heat of the moment, it is often simply unavailable to us, no matter how clearly we can articulate in the abstract what we think needs to happen. There are no principles to guide us here. Often enough there are only metaphors, metaphors that we consult in our efforts to construct a personally authentic and clinically sound response. Sometimes the path to a new freedom between patient and analyst is invisible until a metaphor opens it, and so the wider the range of metaphors at our disposal, the greater our chances of creating new freedom. Levenkron's article widens the range.

REFERENCES

Benjamin, J. (1990), Recognition and destruction: An outline of intersubjectivity. In: *Relational Psychoanalysis: The Emergence of a Tradition,* eds. S. A. Mitchell & L. Aron. Hillsdale, NJ: The Analytic Press, 1999, pp. 183–200.

———— (1999), Afterword to "Recognition and destruction." In: *Relational Psychoanalysis: The Emergence of a Tradition,* eds. S. A. Mitchell & L. Aron. Hillsdale, NJ: The Analytic Press, 1999, pp. 201–210.

Bromberg, P. M. (1998), *Standing in the Spaces: Essays on Clinical Process, Trauma & Dissociation.* Hillsdale, NJ: The Analytic Press.

Ehrenberg, D. B. (1992), *The Intimate Edge: Extending the Reach of Psychoanalytic Interaction.* New York: Norton.

Kohut, H. (1979), The two analyses of Mr. Z. International *Journal of Psychoanalysis,* 60:3–27.

Mitchell, S. A. (1993), *Hope and Dread in Psychoanalysis.* New York: Basic Books.

———— (1997), *Influence and Autonomy in Psychoanalysis.* Hillsdale, NJ: The Analytic Press.

Modell, A. (1991), The therapeutic relationship as a paradoxical experience. *Psychoanalytic Dialogues,* 1:13–28.

Pizer, S. A. (1998), *Building Bridges: The Negotiation of Paradox in Psychoanalysis.* Hillsdale, NJ: The Analytic Press.

Renik, O. (1993), Analytic interaction: Conceptualizing technique in light of the analyst's irreducible subjectivity. *Psychoanalytic Quarterly,* 62:553–571.

———— (1995), The ideal of the anonymous analyst and the problem of self-disclosure. *Psychoanalytic Quarterly,* 64:466–495.

Slavin, M. O. & Kriegman, D. (1998), Why the analyst needs to change: Toward a theory of conflict, negotiation, and mutual influence in the therapeutic process. *Psychoanalytic Dialogues,* 8:247–284.

Stern, D. B. (2003), The fusion of horizons: Dissociation, enactment, and understanding. *Psychoanalytic Dialogues,* 13:843–873.

Stern, D. B. (2004), The eye sees itself: Dissociation, enactment, and the achievement of conflict. *Contemporary Psychoanalysis,* 40:197–237.

24 East 82nd St.
New York, NY 10028

Enactment as Therapeutic Hand Grenade: How Bursts of Emotional Honesty Can Get a Stuck Treatment Moving Again: Discussion of Holly Levenkron's Paper

JUDITH GUSS TEICHOLZ, ED.D.

In my discussion of Levenkron's article, I consider ways of understanding the patient's therapeutic progress that were not highlighted by the author. Adding my own criteria to Levenkron's definition of enactment, I suggest that what the author labels as enactment might be seen as a last-ditch but successful effort to get patient and analyst out of a stuck and painful place. I explore the interplay of confrontational and nonconfrontational interventions in contributing to cure, and I suggest placing a greater emphasis than did the author, on the intersubjective contexts out of which the patient's troublesome behaviors emerged.

IN LEVENKRON'S COMPELLING NARRATIVE, WE SEE INTERPERSONAL courage in action. Levenkron has presented a case in which the analyst's spontaneous emotional honesty served to crystallize a turning point in the patient's treatment. I admire Levenkron's clinical acuity, but would like to suggest a way of understanding her results that is different from the way she herself has proposed. I would suggest that essential interactions took place in

Judith Guss Teicholz, Ed.D., is a Supervising Analyst and Faculty Member at the Massachusetts Institute for Psychoanalysis and is recently retired from the Clinical Faculty of Harvard Medical School at Massachusetts General Hospital, where she taught in the Departments of Psychology and Psychiatry from 1978–2000.

advance of the pivotal events that Levenkron presents to us, interactions that laid important groundwork for the patient's ability to make constructive use of Levenkron's so-called "enactments." Levenkron herself tells us that she could not have confronted Ali at an earlier point in her treatment. When confrontations work therapeutically, it is because they take place in a certain context, often developed over months or years. For this reason, I shall ask: "What other kinds of interactions took place between Levenkron and her patient to render Levenkron's pivotal enactments curative?"

A Brief Comment on the Concept of Enactment

I agree with Levenkron (and with Renik, 1998) that analytic enactment is ubiquitous and ongoing. When considering the analyst's interpretations, clarifications, confrontations, affirmations, or expressions of affect, we cannot say that one of these modes of analytic participation invariably constitutes more—or less—of an enactment than any of the others. This may mean that, from a theoretical standpoint, it is somewhat problematic to isolate a particular interaction and label it an "enactment." But until we can agree on an alternate term by which to refer to Levenkron's focal interactions with Ali, I shall join Levenkron in referring to them as enactments.

Levenkron defines enactment as the spontaneous expression of repressed or dissociated content. I would add that an action can meaningfully be called an enactment when it is a response to unusual pressure brought to bear on the analyst from internal or external sources and entails a content area or intensity of communication that is uncharacteristic for that particular analyst. Because the analyst's motivations for the departure from her own clinical norms remain largely out of awareness, an enactment is often an attempt to arrive at urgent interpersonal goals in a manner that might be unacceptable to the analyst at a more conscious level.

Any analyst is likely to become transiently less available to her patients at times of personal stress, and patients may then react to the analyst's diminished availability with an overwhelming sense of loss and attendant anxiety. An interactive cycle may thus be set in motion with unfamiliar intensities of affect and unaccustomed behavior in both patient and analyst ensuing. In the case under discussion, the patient's demands on the analyst escalated before and after treatment interruptions occasioned by medical and marital crises in the analyst's personal life. This context for the patient's unwelcome behavior is important, and I shall return to it shortly.

Levenkron labels as enactment an episode of sleepiness as well as an instance of (understandable) irritation in response to her patient's insistent demands on her at moments of crisis in Levenkron's life. Although any analyst might doze off momentarily under conditions of stress and exhaustion, or feel irritated in reaction to the kinds of assaults that Ali made on Levenkron, there is unique potential in what the analyst does following such incidents. What Levenkron did was to offer interpersonal feedback to her patient, explaining how aspects of the patient's behavior had contributed to the analyst's unusual feelings and their expression. Levenkron believed that the interpersonal explanation of her own emotional response would give the patient an increased sense of personal agency. More specifically, her explanations were intended to help Ali understand that if she could just refrain from demanding love from the other, she would be more likely to get what she longed for, both from the analyst and in her extratransference relationships. Ali's troublesome behavior subsided in the wake of these interactions, and Levenkron feels that the analysis was moved forward to a deepened level of intimacy.

The Analyst's Expression of Negative Affect as a Prelude to Disruption and Repair

I believe that curative factors not mentioned by Levenkron may have contributed to this happy outcome. In my view, the analyst's direct expression of even mild negative affect holds a potential to disrupt the analytic bond: it can overstimulate the patient, arouse fears of object loss or loss of love, and invoke traumatic memories of more serious failures in self-containment on the part of early caretakers. In spite of these risks, the analyst's modulated expression of negative affect can at certain times help to crystallize a patient's forward movement in treatment. It can have this more positive effect when it follows on a prolonged earlier period during which the analyst has responded more empathically to the patient's provocations. Offered in the context of a reliable empathic bond, the analyst's rare and judicious expression of negative affect can make the analyst feel more real to the patient (Renik, 1998) and therefore more trustworthy (Hoffman, 1998); or it can cut through the historically more repetitive aspects of the treatment relationship to something new.

But to be helpful, the analyst's expression of negative affect must be part of an entire sequence in which the patient may at first become distraught and alienated but is then soothed and contained by re-establishment of the previously lost connection between patient and analyst at a deeper level of understanding. I believe that such a sequence occurred in Levenkron's work with Ali when Ali's initially negative response to an unaccustomed expression of irritation on the part of her analyst was followed by the analyst's interpersonal explanations to Ali. Paradoxically, then, what Levenkron created with Ali seems to be compatible with the Kohutian (1984) notion of disruption and repair, also one of the three principles of salience in the organization of patient–analyst interaction (Lachmann and Beebe, 1996). Allowing for dyad-specific understanding of what might constitute "disruption and repair," I believe that such sequences occurred throughout the material that Levenkron presents to us in which patient and analyst repeatedly lost sight of each other's psychic realities and then found their way back to mutual recognition and empathy.

Enactment as Therapeutic Hand Grenade

Levenkron's focal interactions with Ali also lead me to suggest that an enactment may sometimes be an unconscious but purposeful effort to get beyond a stuck and painful place. As the narrator says in Renata Adler's (1983) novel *Pitch Dark:* "I think when you're truly stuck—when you've stood still in the same spot for too long—you throw a hand grenade into the exact spot where you've been standing, then you jump out of the way and pray." Levenkron's enactments with Ali tended to occur when, in her own words, she felt "stuck, between [her] own boundaries and [her] patient's pain." Her expressions of irritation and interpersonal confrontations may have represented her unconscious but legitimate efforts to get out of that stuck and painful place.

But unlike Adler's narrator—who advocates throwing a grenade and then jumping out of harm's way—Levenkron advises us *not* to jump to our own safety, even after we have set off a minor explosion. She tells us that after we have unwittingly participated in an enactment, we must deliberately remain emotionally present. By her own example she suggests that we follow up the total spontaneity of our enactment with a more intentional communication of our previously unspoken feelings in the relationship. The hope here is that things will be shaken but not destroyed and that in the shaking, they will get moved to a better place.

Of course neither the hope nor the risk of enactment can be consciously assessed in advance since enactments are "now moments" (Stern et al., 1998), cocreated in the turmoil of unidentified intrapsychic and intersubjective influences. Big risks are seldom taken when things are going well in an analysis. They are more often taken after the analyst has tried everything in her usual repertoire and failed. Indeed, Levenkron tells us that she had already tried the "more traditional" ways of speaking to Ali about her destructive envy and had hit a brick wall. I would therefore suggest that many enactments occur when both parties to the dyad have reached a point of last resort and are feeling they must change the status quo or burst. Well, bursting, it turns out, is one way to change the status quo: what I am calling "the enactment as therapeutic hand grenade" is a potentially explosive communication, unconsciously motivated when all else has failed, to get patient and analyst out of a stuck and painful place.

Enactment and the Breakdown of Mutual Recognition

In an earlier version of her article, Levenkron made the point that the most troublesome enactments emerge out of an already ruptured connection in the analytic relationship, associated with failure of recognition. I would therefore suggest that many enactments represent the analyst's unconscious attempt to rectify this failure. Enactments often contain a hidden but potent message: "Please, recognize my existence here; see my point of view!" When it is the analyst who enacts such a plea, it is likely to have followed a long period in which the analyst has been containing, rather than expressing, such feelings. The moment of enactment is the moment when the analyst's previous containing function has broken down under duress. In Levenkron's case, the duress came from what she felt as repeated psychic assaults and impossible demands made on her by her patient.

But to understand an enactment exclusively in terms of the patient's behavior suggests a failure in intersubjective understanding: the patient's assaults may have to converge with moments of the analyst's heightened vulnerability before disruptive enactment becomes inevitable. For instance, I can only imagine that Levenkron's having suffered the twin assaults in her own life of major surgery and marital break-up might have contributed to undermining her more usual tolerance and forbearance in relation to Ali's demands. In any event, since comparable points of vulnerability are likely to emerge in any analyst's life over the course of an open-ended treatment, we must assume that the tendency toward potentially troublesome enactment is ubiquitous. Occasional moments of heightened vulnerability in both patient and analyst lead to a contagion of dysphoric affect that moves quickly away from mutual recognition (Benjamin, 1990) or intersubjective relatedness (Stern, 1985), providing fertile ground for enactment.

In the moment of enactment, the analyst's unfamiliar outburst can push an already vulnerable patient toward rage, compliance, or withdrawal (Winnicott, 1954)—any of these responses might signal a further breakdown of mutuality. An essential task of the postenactment period, therefore, is to re-establish a basis for mutual recognition and empathy. In fact, the difference between an enactment that turns out to be therapeutic, and one that does not, may lie not in the enactment itself but in what the analyst does in the moments and hours after the enactment has been recognized by the two parties to the engagement.

We have earlier noted that following her expression of irritation with Ali, Levenkron explained her behavior by offering interpersonal feedback to her patient that was somewhat confrontational. At first glance, this sequence would seem to violate Levenkron's own theory of intersubjectivity in which she highlights mutuality of both influence and recognition. From the viewpoint of mutual recognition, shouldn't Levenkron have tried to verbalize an understanding of Ali from within the patient's own experience, offering recognition of Ali's feelings in addition to the explanation of her own? And from the viewpoint of mutual influence, shouldn't Levenkron have invited the patient to give an explanation of her behavior that would parallel and complement the analyst's explanations? Shouldn't Ali have been given a chance to say what it was in the *analyst's* behavior or attitude that made Ali feel and behave as she did? The theory of mutual influence would lead us to believe that in any understanding of what was happening in the dyad, the impact of the analyst's words and actions on the patient would be considered on par with how the patient had affected the analyst (Teicholz, 2006).

Interpersonal and Intersubjective Viewpoints

If, however, we believe that such an intersubjective approach to Ali would have been mistaken at these critical moments, then we need to consider how Levenkron did respond—interpersonally rather than intersubjectively—and to account for the fact that the actual mode of interaction seemed to move

Ali's treatment forward, even if it transiently side stepped central principles of the analyst's preferred theory. In my contrasting of interpersonal and intersubjective phenomena here, I use the term *interpersonal* (Mitchell, 1997) to refer to experience between two unique individuals perceived to be acting on the basis of differentiated psyches. I use the term *intersubjective* (Stolorow, Brandchaft, and Atwood, 1987) to refer to experience between individuals perceived to be acting out of permeable and intermingling psyches, exerting continuous mutual influence on one another. For instance, Levenkron tells Ali that it is Ali's demandingness that has led to the analyst's sleepiness or irritation or that has led to Levenkron's inability to give Ali the love she longs for. This message suggests that the buck of interpersonal responsibility stops at the patient's separate psychic doorstep. It does not seem to acknowledge that the responsibility for what happens between patient and analyst might be shared, intersubjectively.

Indeed, Levenkron seems to place a much greater emphasis on what the patient contributes to the analyst's experience than on what the analyst contributes to the patient's, an approach that is more interpersonal than it is intersubjective. Although Levenkron has told us earlier that to achieve the desired goal of intersubjectivity each partner must give up the "tight hold" on her own subjectivity and "directly validate" the other's subjectivity, it would seem that at critical moments she has done almost the opposite: she has held on tightly to her own subjectivity, putting forth her own experience rather than validating that of her patient.

At this point I would like to offer my own explanation of these apparent contradictions. First I would like to say that Levenkron's clinical behavior is completely understandable to me in light of Ali's provocations. What I am questioning is not her clinical actions but rather her representation of them as intersubjective, especially in the sense of mutual recognition. I believe that inevitably Levenkron threw recognition to the winds at certain agonizing moments, in order to get out of a stuck and painful place. Before she could begin to re-establish mutual recognition with Ali, she had to shake off what she was feeling as a death grip on the treatment relationship, coming from Ali's unyielding insistence on one-way recognition for herself alone. While the analyst's *goal* was mutual recognition, because Ali had been demanding continuous *one-way* recognition up to that point, Levenkron was finally moved to insist that Ali consider the analyst's experience, as well. This was probably a matter of Levenkron's psychic survival as an analyst, and the survival of the treatment as well. I am therefore suggesting that to achieve her intersubjective goals Levenkron had, momentarily, to force recognition of her own viewpoint on Ali, and in so doing she had to depart from mutuality.

Empathy and Confrontation: An Essential Dialectic

There are a few other points around which I would differ from Levenkron—again, in explanatory emphasis more than in action. To my mind, Levenkron seems to underplay several of her nonconfrontational interactions with Ali, giving much less therapeutic weight to them than she gives to the more confrontational ones. For instance, she reports having made several references to Ali's early experience with her primary objects but makes no suggestion that these comments might have been facilitative of analytic process or cure. I see these references to Ali's painful early experience as profoundly empathic and as no less emotionally honest than were the interpersonal confrontations to which Levenkron attributes such curative power. When we are able to fully imagine ourselves into our patient's experience, we can become just as impassioned about what other people have done to the patient as we can about what the patient is doing to us. While I agree with Levenkron that the patient's sense of agency can be increased by learning about the interpersonal impact that she has had on others, it can also be increased by gaining an understanding of the impact that others have had on her—and of how that past experience might be contributing to current feelings and behavior.

I believe that Ali's troublesome behaviors might have faded gradually in the face of her analyst's repeated efforts to help her understand them in terms of her childhood feelings of deprivation or, even more importantly, in terms of the reawakening and exacerbation of the sense of deprivation at times of increased distance or separation from her analyst. If this enhanced understanding, by itself, didn't eventually work to change Ali's behavior, then the analyst might have tried a more integrative message to Ali, trying to bring together the intersubjective and the interpersonal in Ali's past and current life. Unwieldy and longwinded as it is, such a message might have gone something like this: "As a child with your father, you had every reason to demand the love he wasn't giving to you. It was your birthright, and he was depriving you of it. And of course your feelings of deprivation are still with you—especially at times like this, when our meetings have been (or are about to be) disrupted. I know that the demands you make on me come from your loneliness and despair. But right now, I'm afraid they're actually getting in the way of my being able to give you what you ask. It's understandable that these feelings would be at their worst right now, just before (or just after) a big separation between us." I would imagine that many of the components of such an intervention had already been suggested by Levenkron in various communications with Ali before the pivotal confrontations that she describes. These less confrontational communications probably worked, together with the pivotal confrontations, to further Ali's treatment in ways not explicitly acknowledged by Levenkron.

Let me offer examples from the material provided us of what I am labeling as nonconfrontational intervention. At one point, Ali reacted to an impending separation by expressing longings to merge with her analyst—to enter and live inside her analyst's body. Although Levenkron felt intruded on by the intensity of her patient's longings, she managed to sustain an empathic position when she said to Ali, "No one showed you that you could be safe even if you were separate. I think your mother showed you the opposite" or a little later, when she said, "No one ever separated from you in a loving way."

I would characterize these communications as empathically conveyed analytic reconstructions (Ornstein and Ornstein, 1980, 1985) that offered essential understanding of Ali's otherwise overwhelming feelings in the here-and-now relationship. I think that Levenkron might have gone even further in this direction, seeking out current triggering events for Ali's difficult feelings and behaviors—making mention, for instance, of the unavoidable but sudden disruptions in Ali's treatment. Ali's feelings of anxiety and loss concerning these events surely contributed to the very behavior on her part that Levenkron was working to change. I believe that the analyst's repeated efforts to explain them, both in terms of Ali's early experience and in terms of the here-and-now, might have been at least as effective in promoting change in Ali's behavior and moving the treatment forward as were the interpersonal confrontations Levenkron describes.

Interpersonal Responsibility

Based on experience with one or two patients I have worked with who remind me of Ali, I imagine that my reactions to Ali would have been quite similar to Levenkron's. But I do not agree with Levenkron (or with Renik, whom she cites) that the analyst's statement of "where she is coming from" necessarily constitutes an act of taking responsibility for the analyst's own behavior. The analyst may well feel that where she is coming from is a reaction to the patient's behavior, but patients often experience such interpersonal feedback as being blamed for the analyst's feelings. They are more likely to experience the analyst as taking responsibility for her feelings when the analyst simply acknowledges them but avoids explaining them in terms of the patient's behavior and attitudes.

Levenkron writes that enactments involving mutual recognition can expand the range of subjective content. I would agree but would add as well that the converse is also true: when enactments do *not* involve mutual recognition, they can *narrow* the range of subjective content—sometimes even bringing analytic exploration to a halt. I think that Levenkron's case material includes both examples of interactions characterized by mutual recognition and by its absence. For instance, when Levenkron feels intruded on by Ali's longings but still manages to understand Ali in the context of her early experience, the analyst is living up to her own ideals of mutual recognition. By contrast, Levenkron's messages of interpersonal feedback to Ali move away from mutuality, attributing as she does her own irritability to Ali's demands. Fortunately, however, Ali took the feedback to mean that her analyst cared enough to step out of her usual role and convey something true, spontaneous, and personal about the impact that Ali was having on her. My only concern, therefore, would be that Levenkron remain alert for later signs that this response might have constituted more of a subtle behavioral compliance on Ali's part than a deep and lasting change of heart and mind.

Certainly if Levenkron's confrontations had not been interwoven and balanced with other kinds of interventions, they might have led to a less positive outcome. In Hoffman's (1998) critical dialectic, any mode of communication can lose its effect if it is used exclusively or routinely. For Hoffman, it is the dialectical tension, *between* ritual and spontaneity—or, I would say, between empathy and confrontation—that lends power to the analyst's pivotal messages. So although Levenkron wrote this article to show us how the emotional honesty involved in certain confrontations served to move a treatment forward, I would wonder if those interpersonal confrontations—however pivotal—were the exceptional intervention in Ali's treatment, rather than the rule. I would imagine that they occurred against a backdrop of Levenkron's equally powerful and compassionately conveyed analytic (re)constructions concerning Ali's formative relationships, many of which were included in Levenkron's report but were not singled out as curative.

Pathways to Mutual Recognition

In the period of treatment that Levenkron has described, her patient seemed to be clinging to a demand for one-way recognition, recognition for herself alone. As is often the case, Ali's demandingness emanated from a child-hood history of painful relationships. Levenkron understood this. But because Ali had not responded to the analyst's more traditional interventions, Levenkron finally saw no alternative but to *force* Ali's recognition, only, however, after long periods of tolerating its absence.

While gentle interpersonal coercion can be one effective last resort in a treatment, there are multiple pathways to mutual recognition in normal development. Children are most likely to grow up recognizing the needs of others when their own needs have been adequately attended to, when, that is, their exposure to parental needs and desires has occurred in small and manageable doses against a larger background of the caretakers' reliable self-containment and selective self-expression. By contrast, parents whose own separate realities are constantly and too much with them—and who thereby expose their children to overwhelming doses of adult affect and desire—may contribute to the development of children who must at an early age adaptively insulate themselves against the needs and affects of others. As adults, they may arrive for treatment quite incapable of mutual recognition; their own subjectivity or sense of self is too compromised, and they have been traumatized by exposure to too much, too soon of their parents' subjectivities.

Most patients who demand one-way recognition, as Ali did, tend to have grown up with their needs for recognition unmet. They have suffered premature and enforced contact with too much of their parents' separate and painful psychic realities. For these reasons, with such patients my intent (not always realized of course) is to share my psychic reality only selectively, attempting to contain my feelings of negative affect.

The work of Beebe, Lachmann, and Jaffe (1997) comes to mind here. They found that children with the most troubled attachments tend also to manifest unusually high-tracking behavior in interaction with their caretakers. These children follow the affect of their caretakers very closely and are distraught when their own affect is not perfectly matched in the relationship. One way to understand Ali's suffocating demands on her analyst, then, is in terms of such a disturbed early attachment pattern and the associated high-tracking behavior that would predictably be exacerbated around her analyst's absences and returns. Additionally, because the analyst's affective self-expression inevitably tends to distinguish her in the patient's mind as a differentiated other, patients with disturbed attachment patterns may also react with pain and rage when the analyst simply reveals her own unique affective responses to the patient. Especially when the analyst's unusual outspokenness occurs around impending absences, and the patient experiences the message as distancing, the negative impact may expand exponentially. Such a sequence might be understood to have occurred between Ali and Holly.

The Analyst's Self-Expression and Self-Containment

For all these reasons and more, I see confrontation and explicit affective honesty as essential but elective elements within a large and flexible analytic repertoire. The analyst must be prepared to be either selectively self-expressive or selectively self-contained—to be affectively open or to hold her feelings until a more efficacious moment occurs for self-expression. Especially when an impasse has been born of the analyst's unusual affective honesty in the first place, the analyst might initially move in the direction of greater affective containment, at least until the rawness of the enactment has had time to heal in both partners.

Interpersonal Feedback versus Intersubjective Context

There is one more area in which I would question Levenkron's emphasis in describing her work with Ali. To my mind, she highlights Ali's *behavior* with too little emphasis on the *context* in which both behavior and feeling arose (Stolorow and Atwood, 1992). For instance, Ali's abusiveness seems to have worsened in the context of hurt feelings, sensual overstimulation, and separation anxiety. Ali's vulnerabilities were such that she was overstimulated by being in proximity to the sight of Levenkron's legs as the two were going up the stairs. Although any analyst might be angered by Ali's false accusation of deliberate seduction, the analyst might later have linked Ali's mistaken accusation and her probable overstimulation at the time. From this contextual vantage point, Ali's experience of the sexual feelings and intentions as coming from outside herself in the form of her analyst's seductive intent could be understood as an unconscious attempt to shield herself from what she would otherwise have felt as her own shameful flooding of desire. These more contextual explanations might have brought

Ali's attention to her off-putting behaviors just as surely as the confrontations did but might also have helped her to place her behavior in the relational situations—and intrapsychic contexts—that had elicited it. I believe that understanding the contextual triggers for a patient's behavior is yet another way to increase the patient's sense of agency—a treatment goal for Ali to which Levenkron herself aspired.

I turn now to Ali's destructive envy—particularly its flare-ups in the face of the analyst's impending absences. Continuing to look at the situation contextually, we might say that when under dread of loss, Ali tended to become more envious and abusive toward Levenkron than at other times. But in Levenkron's actual response to Ali's envy, she often places greater emphasis on its interpersonal impact than on its possible intersubjective triggers. She did not ask, either silently or aloud: "What has exacerbated Ali's despairing or rageful feelings in relation to me just now?"

I have also found it useful to explore the links between a patient's envy on the one hand and her sense of deprivation and damage on the other. It is often a sense of personal deficit that keeps envy alive. If a treatment awakens hope in the patient that her sense of deprivation and damage will be reversed, there is likely to be a spontaneous remission of destructive envy. I believe that people do not usually destroy in others what they believe might someday be theirs. Levenkron herself suggests that what calmed Ali down in the end was hearing that her analyst *wanted* to give her the love that she had been demanding.

Laying the Groundwork for Confrontation

Although in psychoanalysis it can be a good thing to call a spade a spade, I do not think that it was Levenkron's confrontation of Ali that helped Ali to feel less envious. The therapeutic result more probably came through the previous months of treatment in which Ali was gathering imperceptibly within herself the wherewithal to make changes in her life. Ali was able to let go of the envy and its self-defeating behavioral accompaniments only when she had been able to take in enough from the ongoing relationship with her analyst to begin getting what she wanted in her own life. I would guess that prior to the period of treatment that Levenkron describes to us, she had consistently provided for Ali greater understanding and acceptance of Ali's difficult behaviors. I have already pointed to Levenkron's frequent explanations of Ali's feelings in terms of Ali's early relational experience, even in the period of treatment that Levenkron has described to us.

When an analyst participates in an enactment, she has often been extending analytic acceptance to her patient for months on end, even in the face of behaviors that regularly destroy relationships in the patient's extratransference life. I am therefore arguing that diverse analytic phenomena had laid important groundwork for the more confrontational events to which Levenkron attributes curative power. I conjecture that without a fuller accounting of these, her so-called enactments appear to be more instrumental to change in Ali's treatment than they really were.

It is possible that Levenkron brought us into this narrative at a point when both partners were quite ready for change. Ali's need for her old defensive postures may have already been greatly diminished as a result of the ongoing therapeutic action. She was probably sick of her old ways. And Levenkron had probably already been containing both her own and her patient's painful affect for about as long as any analyst could be expected to bear it. Her intuition may have told her that she could let go at this very juncture—a time at which, as we have already noted, many other forces converged that also contributed to a loosening of Levenkron's ordinary reserve.

In an earlier version of her article, Levenkron mentioned that she could never before these critical moments have been so honest with Ali. She wrote that she was able to take the interpersonal leaps that she did only because Ali had already turned a corner in her treatment. I am saying that this corner had been turned by virtue of the richly variegated work that patient and analyst had been doing together over the prior years of treatment. In the earlier clinical work, confrontation and interpersonal feedback may have played a smaller role than they did in this later period of treatment Levenkron has described to us here.

Earning the Right to Emotional Honesty

Every analyst would do well to emulate Levenkron in her affective honesty. But especially when emotional honesty involves confrontation is its timing essential. Levenkron herself tells us that the analyst must *earn the right* to speak so honestly with a patient. I believe that Levenkron earned this right with Ali in many interactions that she described but did not specifically point to as curative, interactions in which Levenkron expressed understanding and acceptance of Ali's difficult behavior, sometimes through reconstruction of Ali's painful early experience and sometimes through other kinds of nonconfrontational messages.

Although I agree with Levenkron that the analyst's emotional honesty is a central part of every successful treatment, I believe that confrontation and interpersonal feedback work in conjunction with other essential modes of relating and do not stand alone among psychoanalytic approaches. Even more importantly, confrontations and interpersonal feedback do not have a monopoly on emotional honesty. Emotional honesty is just as likely to be a central component of affective resonance, analytic reconstruction, and interpretive statements of understanding.

The analyst makes conscious and unconscious choices about which of her selves she shall lead with at any point in her work with a given patient (Teicholz, 1999, 2000, 2001). Levenkron has given us a lively and admirable account of how she used her emotionally honest, outspoken, and assertive selves to facilitate a particular patient's growth at several well-selected moments in a long-term, open-ended, analytic treatment. We have also seen that there were many moments in Ali's treatment when the analyst spoke in more interpretive and empathic tones—when she led with a different analytic self. I have suggested that Ali's ability to use Levenkron's confrontations therapeutically was the result over many months of treatment of Levenkron's broad and flexibly employed repertoire of nonconfrontational as well as confrontational modes of participating in that analytic dyad.

REFERENCES

Adler, R. (1983), *Pitch Dark*. New York: Bantam Doubleday.

Beebe, B., Lachmann, F., & Jaffe, J. (1997), Mother–infant interaction structures and pre-symbolic self and object representations. *Psychoanal. Dial.,* 7:133–182.

Benjamin, J. (1990), An outline of intersubjectivity: The development of recognition. *Psychoanal. Psychol.,* 7 (Suppl.):33–46.

Hoffman, I. Z. (1998), *Ritual and Spontaneity in the Psychoanalytic Process: A Dialectical–Constructivist View*. Hillsdale, NJ: The Analytic Press.

Kohut, H. (1984), *How Does Analysis Cure?* ed. A. Goldberg & P. Stepansky. Chicago: University of Chicago Press.

Lachmann, F. & Beebe, B. (1996), Three principles of salience in the organization of the patient–analyst interaction. *Psychoanal. Psychol.,* 13: 1–22.

Mitchell, S. (1997), *Autonomy and Influence*. Hillsdale, NJ: The Analytic Press.

Ornstein, P. & Ornstein, A. (1980), Formulating interpretations in clinical psychoanalysis. *Int. J. Psycho-Anal.,* 61:203–211.

_____ & _____ (1985), Clinical understanding and explaining: The empathic vantage point. In: *Progress in Self Psychology, Vol. 9,* ed. A. Goldberg. Hillsdale, NJ: The Analytic Press, pp.143–157.

Renik, O. (1998), Getting real in analysis. *Psychoanal. Q.,* 67:566–593.

Stern, D. (1985), *The Interpersonal World of the Infant.* New York: Basic Books.

_____, Sander, L., Nahum, J., Harrison, A., Lyons-Ruth, K., Morgan, A., Bruschweiler-Stern, N., & Tronick, E. (1998), Noninterpretive mechanisms in psychoanalytic therapy: The something more than interpretation. *Internat. J. Psycho-Anal.,* 79:903–922.

Stolorow, R., Brandchaft, B., & Atwood, G. (1987), *Psychoanalytic Treatment: An Intersubjective Approach.* Hillsdale, NJ: The Analytic Press.

_____, _____, & _____ (1992), *Contexts of Being.* Hillsdale, NJ: The Analytic Press.

Teicholz, J. G. (1999), *Kohut, Loewald, and the Postmoderns: A Comparative Study of Self and Relationship.* Hillsdale, NJ: The Analytic Press.

_____ (2000), The analyst's empathy, subjectivity, and authenticity: Affect as the common denominator. In: *Progress in Self Psychology,* ed. A. Goldberg. Hillsdale, NJ: The Analytic Press, pp. 33–53.

_____ (2001), The many meanings of intersubjectivity and their implications for self-disclosure. In: *Progress in Self Psychology, Vol. 17,* ed. A. Goldberg. Hillsdale, NJ: The Analytic Press, pp. 9–42.

_____ (2006). Qualities of engagement and the analyst's theory. *IJPSP,* 1:47–77.

Winnicott, D. (1954), Withdrawal and regression. In: *Through Paediatrics to Psycho-Analysis.* New York: Basic Books, 1975, pp. 255–261.

127 Mt. Auburn Street
Cambridge, MA 02138
judy_teicholz@yahoo.com

Epilogue: Love (and Hate) With the Proper Stranger: Meditation on Change

Ali: I am coming to you for help, but don't tell me anything I don't want to know. I don't really want to change—I just want you to make me feel better. Change is for you, Holly—leave me alone.

(Holly heard—so for now you want to be inside me, not to argue with you, to be molded by you, to be available to you, to be completely at your service.)

Holly: But you say you are in pain and you want a different life. I want you to believe you can change. But if you refuse to change, you will remind me of someone I loved who didn't want to change and it came to a sad end.

(Ali heard—so you won't give me what I want.)

THESE MADE UP SENTENCES REPRESENT THE MOST POWERFUL unconscious agendas through which Ali and I organized our interactions with each other, painful agendas of hope, connection, and loss through which we related. We each wanted the other to do something. Ali wanted me to love her unconditionally and to help relieve her pain; and I wanted to be helpful to someone who was in pain. I discovered that something fundamental in me wanted her to recognize that she needed to change. Because our pain and desires were unconsciously somewhat at odds, Ali and I often entered into clashes such as those represented in my article. These, then, were the conflicts that we brought into the room with us.

One of the interesting tensions underlying several of the discussions of my article is the examination of different paradigms of relatedness and the relationship of these paradigms to "conflict", unconscious or nonconscious. Another tension is organized around meanings of the use

279

of confrontation and self-disclosure and the relevance of these meanings to change. Yet, a third tension concerns enactment of both interpersonal and historical experience and its relationship to dissociation, as well as the relevance of the concept of enactment. At the heart of all the discussions is the unraveling of different notions of intersubjectivity, which span the interpersonal "declarative" levels of communication to the subsymbolic, implicit levels of motivation. I want to thank the discussants for their extremely thoughtful and thought-provoking essays that offer ideas and alternate versions of how each imagined relating to the particular kinds of clashes that Ali and I encountered. I conceptualize these clashes as the organizing "relational conflicts" in which Ali and I were internally enmeshed and which would have to change in both of us for the treatment to succeed. Such mutual change became the goal of treatment for us both.

But First a Story

Once upon a time, a man called Ivan went to a mystic and asked if he could be sent back to have another chance at his life. "I know I wouldn't make the same mistakes again," the man pleaded. The mystic said that this was impossible, that the man would forget everything and do the same things all over again. Ivan got his wish, only years later to find himself once again in the mystic's parlor pleading to be sent back so he could have one more try at doing things over.

The discussants' contributions pushed me to think further about how I might be able to effect in my own practice what the Russian philosopher P. D. Ouspensky's Ivan Osokin could not achieve in his life. For what is psychoanalysis if not a journey like Ivan's into one's own memory that challenges us to change how we operate as a result of that knowledge? And what is a relational psychoanalysis if not a journey of two people involving each other in their pasts and present? A journey into awareness about what has happened and become known as a result of their meeting that might influence the way they make their mutual and separate futures? I will not attempt to address these rich and provocative responses in great detail, nor will I, like Ivan, attempt now to do it differently. Instead, I will provide a very brief meditation on what my work with Ali, the writing about that work, and the responses to it have taught me about change and about the rich and shifting complexities in practicing relational psychoanalysis.

The Relational Unconscious

Barbara and Stuart Pizer focus on how all analysts and patients are influenced by their past histories and how we configure "being with another" through those experiences. They beautifully trace a piece of my own painful and unconscious narrative in Ali's treatment, for Ali's refusal to change mirrored my own mother's resistance to change. Ali's intolerance to loss also mirrored my mother's inability to deal with loss. These ghosts haunted the treatment room and the termination. Ali had a continuous fear that I would die, and I had a continuous belief that she did not want to change. Unbeknownst to me then, there occurred a different outcome than I could have predicted. In stark reality life drew us away from Ali's treatment toward a medical emergency to which she would have to devote herself. We stayed in touch and she went on to battle a deadly illness with bravery and with drive that was built of hope. That hope was required to survive and to do the next piece of work to save her life. I saw in her the very feistiness that was initially reflected through her envy turn into the thing necessary to keep her going and help her to make new meaning in her life.

This outcome differed markedly from my own internalization of a frightened mother who would not take her life in her own hands in order to change. It differed too, from the Ali who was so dependent on others for holding her pain. The one piece I didn't make a point about in my article was the way Ali put most things outside of herself. The pain was outside, located in and mitigated by others who refused to give her what she wanted. In the end she took the pain back inside of herself and dealt with it like a champion. We don't always get the chance to understand the impact on a pattern of treatment or a separation until it has time to evolve in that person's life and is tested by new experience.

History and Relational Critiques

My early experiences as an analyst contradicted arguments that the analyst who is forthright, self-revealing, and interpersonal is simply INTERACTING, rather than using his or her mind/creativity theories to

help the patient. In 1998, when this article was first accepted for publication I had just begun to clarify for myself what I believed a relational
treatment needed to address: that so-called "enactments" and disclosures
are central to effective treatment. However, I was hearing that an analyst
cannot "think" in a field of heightened emotions and that displays of affect are irresponsible when they come from the analyst. But I knew that
an affective presence and self-disclosure were central to my work and to
my idea of relatedness and that patients seemed to get better when I
made fuller use of myself in the process. I believed that more than just
"interacting" was occurring. I also knew, especially with difficult cases,
that an open and honest treatment could not succeed if it didn't contain
compassion and love for one's patient. I approached the writing of this
treatment in an effort to understand for myself and to articulate for others
the therapeutic action in the relational analytic perspective out of which it
evolved. The fact that these arguments remain active and unsettled, as
can be seen in the texts of some of the discussions included in this issue,
attests to their continuing relevance eight years later.

Enactment

What would have had to change for me that day on the stairs to be able to
have said something like Malcolm Slavin's analyst X did when she hypo-
thetically stated, "Look Ali, maybe you're actually sensing something in
me when you say I wanted you to look at my legs, something that goes beyond what I'm aware of. But, as I think about it, it feels to me that maybe
what you're getting at is how much you want to feel that what I feel for you
is real and that I really welcome your passion in seeing me, feeling for me."
And how could I have been more able to disclose something helpful as
Owen Renik catches in my own transference reactions—which often cata-
pulted me into dissociated states—something that prevented me from
"wondering out loud" in some way whether I had been flirting with Ali.
Renik's and Slavin's responses to this vignette helped me to realize that I
was facing several questions at that early stage of the treatment and, in a
sense, in my life: What would have to change in *me* to do this? Who would I
have to be? Was the patient asking me to change something in order to help
her move, rather than only reflecting her narcissistic strivings? What was
she tacitly asking me to do relationally with her and for her to help her?

And, following Philip Bromberg: Can there be intersubjectivity during enactments where dissociation is prominent?

Renik reminds me that the use of the word "enactment" is complex. He explains how I both agree with him that everything can be seen as enactment and yet continue to use the word to describe mental process. Certainly too many authors continue to ascribe different meanings to the word. I was not yet ready to put the word to rest—especially in relation to one focus that Renik had implied: the focus of the relationship of enactment to intersubjectivity and, I would add, the focus of the relationship of enactment to dissociation. For me these two relationships describe the fulcrum between classical and postclassical thinking.

Intersubjectivity

Slavin provides an excellent description and comparative inquiry into the differences, as he sees them, in the two most comprehensive psychoanalytic models of intersubjectivity: the developmental intersubjectivity of Jessica Benjamin (1988, 1995) and the systems version of Robert Stolorow et al. (1974). (I footnote Benjamin's as the predominant intersubjective theory reflected in my work.) As I see it, Slavin is considering—and perhaps coupling—my interest in confrontation as synonymous with a type of "conflict-based" model of relatedness, a model, Slavin interprets, that is like Benjamin's. Such a model of relatedness would likely address inevitable power operations with predictable struggles for positions of dominance. The goal of such a model would be to transcend these power operations in order to reach positions of mutual recognition of each other's, and one's own, separate subjectivities. I believe James Fosshage has described a similar depiction of my use of Benjamin's theory. In fact, this is how I think her theory is generally regarded.

Both Fossage and Slavin raise concern for holding a theory that contains a vision of human relatedness—*as I think they see me illustrating it*—that is fundamentally grounded in power operations. Fosshage, in fact, interprets my intersubjective stance, along with other relational contributors, as "inherently adversarial." I believe this interpretation of the relational perspective is far too narrow; moreover, I don't believe that in my work with Ali I was exclusively tied to seeing motivation through this perspective. Whether or not I want to argue against this as my general mode of organization, I think Slavin and Fossage raise very important considerations. Because of the concern Slavin raises he tries to imagine a different analytic response that provides a different kind of developmental scene. He is not disagreeing with the need to disclose and to provide the patient with a view into the analyst's mind and feelings; nor is he questioning the prevalence of relational conflict; rather, he is looking for alternative organizing principles that might allow a similar type of "affective honesty", without the relational construct of "confrontation" as a requirement for therapeutic action. Slavin is questioning the utility of what I illustrate as "confrontation."

I think that both Slavin and Fosshage, while acknowledging the interpersonal intense shifting attunements that culminate in a successful treatment with Ali, are asking if a theoretical model—one that they see organized around power operations—might be obfuscating the analyst's vision, empathic understanding, and even compassion: If a given relational psychoanalytic model is founded in "the transcending of struggles for dominance," where is there room in it for any other areas of development or systems of motivation? Further, Slavin postulates, wouldn't enactments be different for the analyst who does not see relationship through power operations?

Paradigms of Relatedness

One interesting tension that I made note of in the introduction to this article regards the way Slavin, Fosshage, and Bromberg examine different paradigms of relatedness. What Bromberg is offering is not grounded in a set model for motivation or development. In an exquisite description of his theory of human interaction and enactment, he constructs a different model of the mind in which, he says, there are "… two discreet modes of information processing." I see this as occurring regardless of the motivational systems that are operative. He explains, "The first, the 'subsymbolic' (Bucci, 1997a, 1997b, 2001, 2002) is organized at the level of body experience as 'emotion schemas' relationally communicated through enactment; the second, the 'symbolic,' is organized at the level of language and conflict." These implicit and explicit communications are particular to and coconstructed within each interaction, defining conflict on the "implicit" level as what I have been calling *"relational conflict."* Here we can see how multiple levels are accessed through "interacting."

In Bromberg's model—from which I drew heavily in understanding this case—relatedness is not understood through power operations. It embodies a shifting narrative wherein safety and protection of attachment bonds effect dissociated states and the ability to establish certain types of relatedness. The analytic goals are different. Therapeutic action is influenced by understanding power operations when that is relationally relevant. Intersubjectively, what is sought is the achievement of the capacity for a type of negotiation that prompts shifts out of dissociated states, helping both patient and analyst reach states of relatedness that allow for, in Bromberg's language, interpersonal re-experiencing of what had before been unspeakable. In this perspective, the aim of achieving a mutual, "affectively honest" relationship is central to helping the patient to access information previously dissociated and heretofore able only to be enacted. Making something speakable is not *resolution* of conflict; it is the ability to hold and examine the experience of *relational conflict* as it occurs interpersonally so it can get analytically processed, reflected on and symbolized.

Implicit Communication

Bromberg and Slavin offer ideas that coalesce into another interesting psychoanalytic tension. They both look at "implicit knowledge" and implicit communications. According to the Boston Change Process Study Group, implicit knowledge not only contains fundamental "procedural" knowledge (how to do things like ride a bicycle, etc.) but also contains fundamental knowledge about "being with another" (BCPSG, 1998). Slavin cautions us against relying on "implicit communications"; as such, implicit communications are incomplete representations of our understanding. Slavin is not imagining a "traditional" interpretation when he cautions us against relying only on the "procedural." He is aware of the evocative power (as well as the limitations) of implicit communication; but he also warns us that, however vivid (and representative of what is going on in our coconstructed unconscious) such communications are, valorizing the implicit over the explicit can be problematic. To exemplify his meaning, Slavin creatively rethinks some of my statements, posing them in what he describes as their "explicit" developed form.

I see this re-phrasing as Slavin's attempt to maximize his understanding of another's subjective experience by what I would call "extending the implicit" into consensually validated (Sullivan, 1950) form. One caveat is that overly describing one's own or one's patient's experience can diminish contact by getting us too much in our heads and limiting what Alan Shore calls "right brain to right brain" communication (2003)—the very thing I see enhanced by "affectively honest" communication.

Confrontation

In Bromberg's way of working, confrontation is not thought of as "intrusive." He elaborates the concept of confrontation by summarizing my thinking in the following way: "Being candid is a natural part of negotiation; it is not the application of a technical procedure that is implemented by 'telling it like it is.'" And he adds, "In the process of negotiated confrontation, the two partners learn that their confrontations do not lead to their breaking apart, allowing the patient to more and more safely trust the reliability of a previously repudiated reality—that relational ruptures can be reparable." Tronick and Weinberg (1997), Kohut (1984), Beebe and Lachmann (1994), and other self psychologists see this repair process as the very essence of psychoanalytic treatment. In a more existential way, I often think of Irwin Hoffman's (2000) idea of confrontation as a way to present "ambiguity" to another. Rather than an aggressive mode of communication, then, it can offer other means to grapple with something in your (or in their) mind. Ali had difficulty tolerating ambiguity; looking back, I conclude that this is one of the things that had changed for us.

Stern also has a different reaction to expressions that enter into a particular type of confrontation, as well as to Benjamin's ideas of struggle: "The special kind of confrontation opened up by what Levenkron calls 'affective honesty' is Levenkron's contribution to our understanding of what it takes to shift the struggles for domination that make up enactments into something different, something more like two people each recognizing the other's separate subjectivity (Benjamin, 1990), even if neither likes what they see."

Bromberg also focuses his attention on the clinical use of self-disclosure. We fully agree on how the analyst's self-revelation "in establishing a climate of affective honesty," has an integral place in relational therapeutic action. He describes the "action" in self-revelation as creating "... a transitional reality [that] can begin to take shape between patient and analyst that has room for the subjective experience of each partner and space for relational negotiation that is really alive." This work allows for the development of a fuller and deeper type of exchange and allows for the integrated mutual holding (not resolving) of conflict. He highlights my statement that the "analyst's ability to do this with someone has to be earned," and feels earning this "climate" evolves from the ongoing "struggle the analyst has with his own limitations" and from revisiting negotiations. (For a fuller discussion of this subject see Bromberg, *Awakening the Dreamer,* 2006.)

Authenticity and Coconstruction

I think the difference in the way Stern views my approach lies in his own notions of coconstruction, and unformulated experience, and in the way he interprets the relationship between dissociation and enactment, all of which he has written about at length elsewhere (2004). Here he adds, "It has been clear to relational and interpersonal analysts for a number of years now that, in each moment, we have no choice but to select one of the personal responses available to us … there is no objective 'platform' (Mitchell, 1997) or 'perch' (Modell, 1991) on which it is possible for the analyst to retreat from subjectivity. The process of selecting which of these personal responses to employ is understood by most of these analysts to be a search for the analyst's authentic responsiveness to the patient; But which authenticity? …How should the analyst make her selection?"

Stern affirms that "affective honesty" has a particularity. It is not as simple as an honest show of feeling and "cannot be generated at will." "Affective honesty is not an algorithm for selecting a clinical response. The idea will help those clinicians for whom it resonates, as it does for me; but the particular shape of affective honesty, and the moments of its appearance, must always be unforeseeable. The analyst never knows when she will find herself suddenly able to destabilize an enactment, and often enough she finds out that she has done so only in retrospect. Even authenticity, that is, is a contextual matter" (Mitchell, 1993, pp. 123–150).

Grenades

I want to stress *my* understanding of the affect expressed during these particular confrontations. It was implicit that I was trying to offer Ali something that she was never offered before. Her aggressive negotiating style had aggravated and provoked her father, who didn't know how to negotiate with the "little tyke" that Ali became in his presence. We had investigated the transferential implications of these parental empathic failures many times. Slavin asked why at one juncture I had reflected to myself that if I had interpreted in a more traditional way I would have lost her. The reasons were twofold. By then I had tried more traditional interpretations with limited success and, in addition, I felt that Ali needed to know that I was there with her, grappling with what she wanted from me, and I felt she needed to know that I wanted to try to give her something, even if I couldn't. I had to find a way to express this. As I remember the feelings when I was with Ali, during those three "confrontations" that I illustrated—even though I am going back over nine years—I remember that I had wanted to offer Ali a series of compromises. I was trying to make certain "deals," which were predicated on what Ali had been telling me all along that she desired—that she very specifically wanted me to show love for her and to give her more. I primarily experienced these "confrontations" as *invitations* to *preserve the treatment and our mutual integrity*. In this sense they were not confrontations in the usual way we think of the concept, but rather a type of holding.

It is always interesting to observe how differently we all read material. For example, Slavin thought that in my "form of a confrontation," I was expressing both my love and hate for Ali and giving her a subjective read on our conflict "as a clash of interpersonal strategies for negotiating affective response." He interprets that in this "form" I was offering Ali a way to shift to a less aggressive negotiating style.

Teicholz's views of intersubjectivity and confrontation are very different from mine. I'm respectful, but also I am puzzled at what seems to be a narrowing of the definition I set out to explain in my approach. Teicholz seems to be identifying intersubjectivity with some of Benjamin's definition that refers to a specific type of mutual recognition. I believe that she misses the evolution I have tried to demonstrate of *negotiated efforts* at experiencing each other and ourselves as separate subjectivities resolving the tensions and clashes between us. I use the word *negotiating* to include the use of empathic appreciation. In these negotiations had I specifically questioned Ali about her reactions to my statements, perhaps Teicholz would perceive the mutual recognition contained in our dialogue as the type of dialogue she is missing. But I did experience the dialogue surrounding these "deals" as explicitly including a shared recognition of each other's limits and capacities. In this case, Ali's style was to freely tell me what she thought of my interventions.

If Teicholz saw my words as grenades, she had to see their effect as explosions. Explosions might seem a metaphor for a much needed destabilization in the treatment, but the metaphor connotes aggression and destruction as well. If the analyst advocates freely expressing her own aggression and destruction that would just be self-indulgent. If it is a matter of the analyst engaging the patient where they are and trying to work at working things out—then they are not throwing grenades. Teicholz complements me for not getting out of the way once the grenades hit the ground—as did the women in the story Teicholz quoted. Incidentally, in my perception Ali didn't give me any reason to think I should have run. With Teicholz holding images such as these, it would seem difficult for a meeting of our minds, either Teicholz's mind and mine or, through Teicholz's conceptualization, Ali's mind and mine. There might only be, as Teicholz implied, Teicholz's appreciation, and even identification, with my "reactions" to Ali. Reading Teicholz's discussion, however, I sincerely appreciate how thoughtful it is. I am also left feeling that Teicholz got situated in something Bromberg mentioned in his discussion: "... [B]ecause of the volatility in the transference–countertransference enactment, using this case etches [Holly's] point in high relief, but it also runs the risk that analysts with leanings toward other schools of thought could choose to read Levenkron's paper as implying that the clinical material is presented as paradigmatic, saying in effect that if affective honesty is to be respected, then relational psychoanalysis is inevitably a process of "living-through" and "working-through" volcanic enactments."

Change

I sometimes take for granted the multiple aspects of a relational sensibility. It is exactly that multiplicity that compelled me to both appreciate all the discussions and also to think about the goals of discourse with such an amalgam of knowledge and ideas. I think we all cannot help but sense certain prejudices in those writers who responded from a more or less Relational/Self Psychological vantage point and, as well, sense the prejudices of those who are more inclined toward responding from as Interpersonal/Relational sensibility. A commonplace within the psychoanalytic community is that the former has been less comfortable with aggression, and the latter, more comfortable with it. I think this is probably true. It's a conversation that began sixteen years ago, *Psychoanalytic Inquiry* (Volume 10, Number 4, 1990) carried a case presentation by James Fosshage, and discussions by several authors including Steven Mitchell. Mitchell's response to that case and Fosshage's response to him contain the seeds of the idea Fosshage expresses in this Issue.

Namely, that a basic organizing principle for many relational analysts is to see human relatedness as fundamentally adversarial, evidenced by their language (e.g., collision of subjectivities) and for many by their adherence to Benjamin's dominance and bondage paradigm. How then, do we avoid being entrenched in stereotypes so that other ideas may have the opportunity to re-shape us?

Fosshage, sixteen years ago, may have been locating this idea in the connection between relational and interpersonal psychoanalysis when, in its origins, interpersonal analysts were often seen as "no-nonsense" analysts who used confrontation in a more adversarial way (see interview of Edgar Levenson, CP, October 2005). While an "empathic stance" was not a tenet of the interpersonal model, empathy began to be addressed as evolving out of the interaction with the patient—out of an effort to understand what is going on between you that is motivating you both to behave in a specific way (Bromberg, 1986). Current thinkers suggest that in the course of working with dissociated material that becomes available from the work done within enactments, we can "move" into reflective thinking that can shift our views to new perceptions of the other—and of ourselves—opening up the possibility for empathic connection and change (Benjamin, 2004; Bromberg, 1986, 2006; D.B. Stern, 1997).

Fosshage is concerned that a focus on power dynamics is the single organizing principle of relatedness in my work with Ali. Relational/interpersonal analysis does attend to power dynamics as one feature of the interaction. However, relational psychoanalysis involves a sensibility, rather than a limited, exacting theory committed to only one way of seeing behavior. The "doer/done to" complementarities in Benjamin's theory (1990) describe an aspect of human nature that struggles with a wish to be seen, known, and accepted, i.e., recognized. The therapeutic action, as Fosshage correctly describes, is to transcend the problem of "otherness" and I would add—from Benjamin's more current writing—the problem of a collapse into what she calls "two-ness" (2004), The goal is in establishing two separate subjectivities, both more capable of negotiation and recognition with another. I agree with Fosshage that there are other forms of motivation, such as affiliation, contribution, camaraderie, and, as Fosshage adds, caretaking. However, I hold to Gerald Stechler's (2003) idea that "pivotal moments in our life experience consist of the negotiation of crises. Our capacity to reorganize around crises is what makes our lives possible, and what makes us human" (p.718). Stechler's last point may indeed reflect Fosshage's differences with putting "power issues" at the center of human experience.

However, Stechler describes a Chinese definition of the word for crisis that combines the characters for "threat" and "opportunity." Accordingly, Stechler says, "negotiating has all the volatility and intensity and resistance to changethat are familiar within more traditional therapy, plus more— more because the negotiating therapist, as contrasted with the interpreting therapist, introduces his or her own affective being into the negotiating process. In the course of intensive therapy the therapist's own being is challenged and open to alteration" (2003). This idea of *negotiated* alteration, for me, better describes relational psychoanalysis than the "adversarial" relationship Fossaghe mentioned above. It is from Stechler's negotiated "alteration" that I would ask Fosshage: How can we be available to the type of shifting Stechler describes? Fosshage's own model, anticipates being able to *consciously* shift or orchestrate moves from one mode of relatedness into another. The work I set out to do with Ali, using an integrative clinical model that privileges affective openness and flexibility contains at its heart an acceptance of shifts in self states, authentic empathic resonance, and what I am calling the work of "intersubjective negotiation."

The Present

What I would say now about motivation is broader than what I said eight years ago when I wrote, after Levenson (1994) and Stechler (2003), that the self is fundamentally motivated by the desire to be desired by the other. I still believe this is a fundamental relational motivation. I would add that what motivates interaction on a micro-organizational level is best put in the way the BCPG (1998, 2005) present it regarding what they are describing as the search, on the procedural level, for what they are calling "fittedness." "It is a process of trying to get closer, or further away, or to avoid something happening, or to get something to happen, or to increase or decrease the state of arousal or to shift the affective state in relation to the other." This procedural, subsymbolic level of motivation appears to be a much simpler model than constitutes the complexities of Benjamin's developmental theory of complementarities or Fosshage's caretaking or self–object relatedness. When we think of the macro level of motivation, I certainly agree with Fosshage, based on his work with Lachmann and Lichtenberg (2001), and Jay Greenberg (1991) that there is more than one type of motivational system. I like the term "modes of mediation" used by Donald Moss (2005). I think it bridges theories of motivation with the variety of clinical applications an analyst might adopt in order to mediate personal strivings, whether for safety, caretaking, or mastery over "who did what to whom." The difference in the application of any idea that requires "state changes," or what Fosshage is calling "shifts in relatedness," is how such changes—shifts in the analyst—might be accomplished in a way that optimizes the process of change.

This work is part of a dialectic process (Hoffman, 1998) that can more or less motivate us to call on or evoke different aspects of ourselves and each other—depending on where our awareness lies in the moment—and refers to what Benjamin calls use of the "third" (2004).

This shifting is part of the work I referred to as "learning" the ability for self-revelation and movement that we can find ourselves experiencing during internal and interpersonal negotiations.

Conclusion

I had the opportunity to speak with Ali several times throughout the last four years that followed the ending of our treatment. We have both gone through a lot over this time period, and our perspectives have changed—but I would bet that unless we both really wanted to have a different experience of our "separate" selves, we could each imagine like Ivan in the beginning of this meditation, a particular event that occurred between us and before it went up into a puff of "memory smoke", picture it happening in the same way but, still, wishing it wouldn't. Triggers are emblazoned and carved in memory. I believe we both came to want something different. So how can we, as Donnel Stern (1997) implies elsewhere, change what we already know? How do I/we reflect on this treatment through what we have learned about the world and about ourselves? That might be what is needed, but that might be the hardest part.

Do we do this then as we sit with, as well as without, our patients? Can patient and analyst be reflective in the moment? I think we can, if we are willing to change some essential part of ourselves that no longer wants/ wishes to have the same self–other experience (Slavin and Kriegman, 1998). In short, we cannot change unless we are open to a different outcome; and I suspect we feel this as relevant within the interaction although this desire is further influenced by the "third" element, most of our theories, our peers, and our responsibilities to our patients. Slavin points to the underlying reflective attitude of hope and a refusal to let go—almost a driving force to return and repeat interactions—in the hope of getting it right this time—but, returning again to Ivan's delemma, we have the potential to know that we are likely not to get it right and that hope lies in the coconstruction of new narratives and perceptions; that is, the hope of that slight connection or slight shift facilitated by the other that can suddenly open a new door. I was willing to try as many different approaches as I could think might work, and this—the returning of hope to what may feel like a dying system or a dead end—is the closest conception I have arrived at to describe "reflectiveness in action." In a moment we feel a different feeling that pulls us toward another effort: We are able thereby to stay connected with our hope and expectations that analysis works.

My work with Ali had an urgent and intense effect on me, as well as her. I am grateful to her for her permission to write about our shared history together, but I am even more grateful for her curiosity, which brought us to a deeper place of friendship and respect. When she first agreed to the publication of this article she asked if she could read it, and I suggested that she do so in my presence. Each session, for several weeks, began with Ali's asking if we could look at the paper again. It was fascinating to her, and as she reread sections, she would ask if that were what had happened. Then we would go over the events again and reconstruct the therapy in a new voice. I felt this period was as healing as the entire analysis. It certainly was for me. We could sit together and talk about what we each perceived in a new way. It was as if she were rewriting with me a newer narrative over the narrative I had constructed in the paper. Would this last narrative be the one we will keep?

REFERENCES

Beebe, B. & Lachmann, F. (1994), Representation and internalization in infancy: Three principles of salience. *Psychoanal. Psychology,* 11(2):127–165.

Benjamin, J. (1988). *Bonds of Love.* New York: Pantheon.

_____(1992), Recognition and destruction: An outline of intersubjectivity. In: *Relational Perspectives in Psychoanalysis,* ed. N. J. Skolnick & S. C. Warshaw. Hillside, NJ: The Analytic Press.

_____(1995), *Like Subjects Love Objects.* New Haven, CT: Yale University Press.

_____(2004), Beyond door and done to: An intersubjective view of thirdness. *Psychoanal. Quart.,* 1:5–46.

Bromberg, P. (1986), The mirror and the mask: On narcissism and psychoanalytic growth. In: *Essential Papers on Narcissism.* Ed. A.P. Morrison. New York: New York University Press, 438–466.

_____(2006), *Awakening the Dreamer: Clinical Journeys.* Hillsdale, NJ: The Analytic Press.

Bucci, W. (1997), *Psychoanalysis and Cognitive Science:A Multiple Code Theory.* New York: Guilford.

Fosshage, J. (1990), Clinical protocol. *Psychoanal. Inq.* 10(4):461–477.

Greenberg, J. (1991) *Oedipus and Beyond.* Cambridge, MA: Harvard University Press.

Hoffman, I.Z. (2000), At death's door. *Psychoanal. Dial.* 10:823–846.

_____ (1998) Ritual and spontanaiety in the psychoanalytic process. In: *Ritual and Spontaneity in the Psychoanalytic Process: A Dialectical Constructivist View.* Hillsdale, NJ: The Analytic Press.

Kohut, H. (1984), *How Does Analysis Cure?* Chicago: University of Chicago Press.

Levenson, E. (1994), Beyond countertransference—Aspects of the analyst's desire. *Contemp. Psychoanal.* 30:691–707.

Lichtenberg, L.D., Lachmann, F., Fosshage, J.L. (1992) *Self and Motivational Systems: Toward a Theory of Psychoanalytic Technique.* Hillsdale, NJ: The Analytic Press.

Mitchell, S.A. (1990), Discussion: A relational view. *Psychoanal. Inq.* 10(4):523–540.

_____ (1993), *Hope and Dread in Psychoanalysis.* New York: Basic Books.

_____ (1997), *Influence and Autonomy in Psychoanalysis.* Hillsdale, NJ: The Analytic Press.

Modell, A. (1991), The therapeutic relationship as a paradoxical experience. *Psychoanal. Dial.* 1:13–28.

Moss, D. (2005), Trophy and triumph/shock and awe: On the clinical power of the Abu Grabe photos. Presented at the winter meeting of the American Psychoanalytic Association. New York: University Forum.

Ouspensky, P. D. (1947), *Strange Life of Ivan Osokin.* New York: Holme Press.

Slavin, M.O. & Kriegman, D. (1998),Why the analyst needs to change: Towards a theory of conflict, negotiation, and mutual influence in the therapeutic process. *Psychoanal. Dial.,* 8:247–284.

Stechler, G. (2003), Affect: The heart of the matter. *Psychoanal. Dial.* 13(5):711–726.

Stern, D.B. (2003), The fusion of horizons. *Psychoanal. Dial.* 13(6):843–873.

Stern, D.N. (1997), *Unformulated Experience: From Dissociation to Imagination in Psychoanalysis.* Hillsdale, NJ: The Analytic Press.

_____ Bruschweiler-Stern, N., Lyons-Ruth, K., Morgan, A., Nahum, J., Sander, L., (1998), Non-interpretive mechanisms in psychoanalytic therapy: The "something more" than interpretation. *Internat. J. Psycho-Anal.* 79:903–921.

_____ _____ _____ _____ _____ & _____ (2005), The "something more" than interpretation revisited: Sloppiness and cocreativity in the psychoanalytic encounter. *J. Amer. Psychoanal. Assn.* 53: 693–729.

Stolorow, R.W., Atwood, G.E., & Ross, J. (1978), The representational world in psychoanalytic therapy. *Internat. Rev. Psycho-Anal.* 5:247–256.

Sullivan, H.S., (1950), The illusion of personal individualtiy. In: *The Fusion of Psychoanalysis and Social Science.* New York: Norton, pp. 198–226.

Tronick, E.Z. & Weinberg, M.K. (1997), In: *Postpartum Depression and Child Development,* ed. L. Murray & P. Cooper. New York: Guilford, pp. 54–81.

Holly Levenkron, L.I.C.S.W.

Editor's Epilogue

It has been a great privilege to serve as editor of this ground-breaking issue comprising a series of relational discussions on Holly Levenkron's compelling case of Ali, in which Levenkron illustrates a relational approach to therapeutic action. I believe this issue offers a unique contribution to our understanding of a relational sensibility. The contributors, all outstanding clinicians in their own right, present alternative views on some of the central organizing concepts inherent in this perspective, including, in no particular order, enactment, confrontation, self-revelation, meaning construction, conflict, negotiation, dissociation, intersubjectivity, recognition, authentic engagement, empathy, and Levenkron's own contribution to relational thought, affective honesty. The issue as a whole thus provides a compendium on relational understanding, complete with an embodiment of the tensions that exist among relationalists as they considered and addressed the same clinical material. As readers, we were able to view the variety of conflicting meanings, assumptions, and consequences of this still-emerging psychoanalytic frame.

In this necessarily short epilogue, I will dip into the discussions of our commentators to illustrate the how relational concepts are described in these contributions. Obviously I can do no more than sample these ideas; the richness of the discussions defies any complex codification of them here.

I'll be able to examine only a few of the relational constructs I listed above, then, and only randomly, considering confrontation, negotiation, intersubjectivity, self-disclosure, enactment, dissociation, and affective honesty, all featured by Holly Levenkron in her clinical material and viewed by her as vitally connected to the therapeutic change illustrated in her work with Ali.

Phillip Bromberg

Beginning with Phillip Bromberg, he asserts that in postclassical analytic work, the analyst doesn't avoid participating in the dyad but, rather, using disclosure as a central part of the process, continuously monitors the effects of her participation to further therapeutic efficacy. Bromberg perceives Holly Levenkron as facilitating intersubjective negotiation with Ali through her nonintrusive self-revelations and her open but safety-preserving confrontations. By talking with Ali about her own complex subjectivity, sharing with her, her own inner experience, as well as, as Bromberg says, her experience of her experience, Holly earns the right to the affective honesty that underlies her openly confrontational stance. Bromberg writes that Holly's affective honesty is balanced by affective safety, however, with her attunement to Ali's safety being experienced from within the relationship rather than being a provision of empathy as a technical stance from the outside.

By applying Wilma Bucci's work on two modes of information processing, symbolic and subsymbolic, Bromberg explains enactment as the means by which subsymbolic emotional schemas can be communicated in treatment. When the individual has experienced trauma, the traumatic events remain unprocessed cognitively. Normal dissociative processes are recruited automatically by the traumatized individual to protect the self from being destabilized by pathological emotional schemas created by such traumatic events. Then, in therapy, such dissociated, pathological, subsymbolic experience is enacted in the dyad, rendering internal conflict, and its resolution, possible through the enactment. The goal of treatment is the better integration of dissociated schemas. Bromberg notes further, in agreement with Levenkron, that the working through of the enactment is not accomplished afterwards but is done within the lived experience with the analyst, citing Bucci's assertion that the activation of dissociated experience in the session itself is central to therapeutic action. Bromberg then asserts that Bucci's research confirms Bromberg's, and Levenkron's, ideas that "the analyst's revealing is part of the relational process through which cognitive control over hyperaroused affective experience is regulated by the patient's self-reflective function … facilitated by the integration of dissociated schemas taking place through subsymbolic experience in the session itself. This allows for cognitive symbolization of experience formerly only enacted, increasing the patient's trust in his ability to think about overwhelming experience...." The analyst, too, contacts a part of the self in the enactment, enabling her to think about what had been discovered through interactive participation. Hence, Bromberg affirms and expands Levenkron's views about the therapeutic value of enactment, confrontation, self-revelation, conflict, negotiation, dissociation, and affective honesty.

Judith Teicholz

Judith Teicholz offers a somewhat different perspective, especially in her view on confrontation, self-revelation, and enactment as they make their appearance in this material as well as their connections to therapeutic action. She sees Levenkron as underplaying her nonconfrontational interactions with Ali that had taken place before the events recorded in Holly's presentation, speculating that earlier in the treatment Holly's profoundly empathic understanding of Ali's childhood experience facilitated the process and the cure, and that these interventions in the treatment were not just empathic but also emotionally honest. For example, Teicholz asserts that it was not Holly's confrontation of Ali that helped to allay Ali's envy. Rather, this therapeutic result came from the previous months of treatment where more empathy was involved. By not describing what came before the confrontations, Teicholz says, the "so-called enactments" seem more instrumental in the treatment than they actually are; in her earlier work with Ali, preceding the material included in her presentation, Holly had used less confrontation and "interpersonal feedback" than was documented in this material. Moreover, Teicholz herself would have done more in the interactions portrayed here to seek out the current triggering events that lay behind Ali's feelings and behavior, carefully establishing the context for what occurred; explaining Ali's feelings and behavior in terms of either past or current triggering events would have been at least as effective, Teicholz asserts, as the interpersonal confrontation illustrated here in the clinical material.

In considering enactment, Teicholz says that an action can be called an enactment when it constitutes an uncharacteristically intense response to internal or external sources; it is an unconscious effort to arrive at urgent interpersonal goals in a manner unacceptable on a conscious level. The analyst's enactive expression of negative affect to the patient's provocations, when it follows on a period of empathic responsiveness to such provocations, can promote the therapeutic process, allowing the analyst to seem real and trustworthy; but such negative responses must necessarily appear in a sequence of disruption and repair, with the analyst's irritation followed by interpersonal explanations, moving toward mutual recognition and empathy. Teicholz sees Levenkron's enactments as an unconscious effort to move Ali and herself beyond a stuck place in the treatment. Holly's enacted message "Please recognize me" followed on a period of Holly's containing her negative feelings in reaction to Ali's assaults. But if the enactment is understood only in terms of Ali's behavior it becomes a failure in intersubjective understanding. Holly's own heightened vulnerability made the enactment inevitable. An essential task of the postenactment period, according to Teicholz, is to reestablish mutual recognition and empathy, with the therapeutic effectiveness of the enactment dependent on what the analyst does following the engagement. Levenkron should have offered feedback from with the patient's experience, showing recognition of Ali's feelings in addition to explaining her own. Moreover, Levenkron should have invited the patient's explanation of the enactment to parallel her own. Mutual influence, she asserts, means that what happens in the dyad is in terms of the effect of the analyst's words and actions on the patient as well as the effect of the patient's words and actions on the analyst. This would establish intersubjective, as opposed to interpersonal, relating—the former a relating between two permeable psyches that are intermingled with continuous mutual influence between them, and the latter a relating between two differentiated individuals without mutual influence.

Teicholz concludes that confrontation and explicit affective honesty must be used selectively from within a large and flexible repertoire with a dialectic existing between empathic and confrontational responsiveness.

Malcolm Slavin

Malcolm Slavin indicates his appreciation for Holly's openness in describing her affective honesty, but he himself does not view confrontation (versus interpretation) as the best way of achieving it; he feels there are other ways of conceptualizing the intersubjective clash with Ali and responding to it that would also have been effective. Levenkron, Slavin writes, uses Benjamin's understanding of intersubjectivity, in which there is an inevitable requirement to transcend the universal dynamics of domination and subjugation. This is distinguished from Stolorow et al.'s intersubjectivity, in which clashes are rooted in the differences in subjective worlds in the dyad and are not necessarily derivatives of relational power dynamics between them. Slavin offers a vision of affective honesty, confrontation, and interpretation in an alternative intersubjective context, wherein a given analyst might also experience Ali as aggressive and also feel that her own subjectivity has been misunderstood. While angry herself, Slavin's putative analyst doesn't see her conflict with Ali as rooted in Ali's counterproductive negotiation but instead in their differing perspectives, their differing ways of organizing their subjective worlds. A response that is not confrontational, but that recognizes Ali's subjectivity and then reframes it, may also be an effective basis for negotiation. This is not a better stance than confrontation, Slavin asserts, but a different way to convey compassion and the patient's impact on the analyst, a way that is more interpretive than enactive, and a way for emotional honesty to also be present, as long as the analyst allows the process to release her from her own subjective world and to reconstruct a new one.

Slavin offers an additional meaning of enactment for the Holly–Ali dyad: a needed enactment of a developmental scenario wherein Ali experiences recognition of something pervading her request for an erotic response as well as for an other who doesn't need his or her subjectivity to either clash or coincide. This is more consistent with Stolorow et al.'s version of intersubjectivity than with Holly's own emphasis on the use of intersubjective clashes in the analytic relationship, especially those that challenge dissociated aspects of the analyst's own identity and, through affective honesty, allow the patient to comprehend her impact on the analyst. Slavin's emphasis is on the enactment that forms around the patient's wanting the analyst to go where she wouldn't go in another relationship. Slavin says analysts are called on to revisit in themselves their own versions of core, human, existential issues; to reopen tensions they have, ostensibly, already resolved; to produce, or share, or bear, some view of themselves that their patients need. Slavin says that to join a patient in her need in this way might seem to violate ourselves, whole tracts of our subjective reality, our analytic role, or the therapeutic frame itself. The patient's apparently coercive tactics might actually entail a vital human need to see who we are and what kind of potentially new experience he or she can have with us. Analysts may have to open their own versions of the same human dilemmas that had proved overwhelming to their patients: lifelong challenges that we can't cease to grapple with. Thus, Slavin sees Holly as having, through her work with Ali, to reopen, revisit, and suffer anew something old in herself—her own genuine, personal conditions for feeling love and hate and loss—thereby creating a level playing field in the developmental enactment between them.

James Fosshage

James Fosshage, too, asserts that intersubjective relatedness is not inherently adversarial, conflictual, and oppositional. He compares his own posi-

tion in this regard with that of Holly Levenkron. Holly, following Jessica
Benjamin's postulate of a constant tension existing between recognizing
the other and asserting the self, conceptualizes intersubjective relatedness
as containing an inevitable collision of realities and colliding of agendas,
requiring that each person surrender some aspect of their hold on reality as
a part of the negotiating process. In contrast, Fosshage views the analyst's
subjectivity as potentially facilitative of his or her comprehension of the
other's subjectivity. Further, he believes that as analysts we must hear, recognize, and implicitly validate the patient's subjectivity to be therapeutically effective. Moreover, not only does he disagree that intersubjective relatedness is necessarily adversarial, but Fosshage suggests that Holly's
focus on intersubjective relatedness in itself overlooks other very important
forms of being with, such as selfobject relatedness and caretaking relatedness. Fosshage thus plays down the role of confrontation in therapeutic action, noting the use of the other for self-regulation, for mirroring, for idealizing, and for twinship as well as for caretaking, based on the empathic
capacity to resonate with affects, to identify with experience, and to understand the needs of the other. These ways of being with the other create, not
conflict in the dyad, but mutually enhancing interaction.

In terms of enactment, Fosshage notes that Levenkron emphasizes the
unconscious, dissociated aspects of both analyst and patient in the interaction and the subsequent conscious awareness as central to her theory of
analytic change. But in his own interactive systems model, everything
that occurs in an analytic encounter is an interaction, with the verbal and
the nonverbal differentiated. He defines enactments as affectively poignant interactions that can be positive or negative and conscious and/or
unconscious.

Owen Renik

Perhaps the most radical position on the concept of enactment is taken by
Owen Renik. He agrees with Levenkron that it is misleading to use the term
to denote a discrete, identifiable moment in the clinical interaction. But he
goes further, arguing in effect that nothing is added to our clinical understanding by using the concept of enactment at all. The term, he says, derives from Freud's mistaken and now discarded idea that thought and motor
action are distinguished from one another and mutually exclusive, and that

if fantasies and constituent motives are acted out they would be unavailable for analysis.

Renik also examines Holly's self-disclosure and its lack in the clinical material. He notes first of all that Ali is on the couch, wondering why a relic from a one-person classical theory based on the necessity for projection onto a blank screen would be used in a therapy such as that between Holly and Ali based in a theory of intersubjectivity. Here the analyst is not best viewed as anonymous but as maximally available to be known by the patient. In this regard, Renik asks of Levenkron, why not tell Ali the reason for her cancellation? In this question, he isn't suggesting that the analyst yield to the patient's curiosity; nor is he denying the analyst's entitlement to privacy of self-interested motives. The reason for Holly's nondisclosure is self-interest, Renik asserts, not Ali's well-being, as Holly seems to suggest. It might have been helpful to Ali to know that Holly had problems too. Holly seems to invoke the value of self-selective anonymity. Renik detects some hints of a traditional authoritative stance covertly present in this relational analysis, but, he says, Holly and Ali did find their way out of the impasse of envy through intersubjecetive exchange and successful negotiation.

Donnel Stern

Donnel Stern, considering the concept of enactment, notes that the substance of Levenkron's view is that as the analyst is never outside of enactment, she cannot wait for it to end in order to deal with it. She must act within the enactment through affective honesty, negotiating between her own desire and that of the patient's. Both the patient and the analyst exert conscious and unconscious influence on the other to recognize and satisfy her own desire. Stern asserts his own view that enactment is engaged desire.

Levenkron's goal in writing her paper was to offer, Stern writes, "an illustration of how the relational principles she admires in the contributions of others might work in practice—her own, very personal kind of practice. The value of the paper lies in its example: it is a way of working for us to consult, in our minds, as we sit with our patients, as we try to work out our own ways of conducting psychoanalytic work."

Stern concludes that "Affective honesty" is Levenkron's original contribution to relational analysis. He views the concept as one of those meta-

phors that can be accessed, while engaged in treatment, when we are looking for help to see and feel what we cannot yet see and feel.

Barbara and Stuart Pizer

Finally I will turn to the contribution of Barbara and Stuart Pizer, who begin their discussion with a consideration of the constructs of enactment,
intersubjectivity, and negotiation. Enactments become intersubjective relating, they write, through negotiation that is intrapsychic as well as relational. This involves the analyst's internal negotiation between her
transferences and her recognition, with a loss of the tension between transference and recognition constituting a breakdown in intersubjectivity. The
Pizers differentiate a bit from Holly's minimizing the importance to the
process of negotiating enactment of the achievement of insight into one's
countertransference. They also amend Holly's stated view that negotiating
enactment toward the achievement of intersubjectivity requires that patient
and analyst each give up their tight holds on their own subjectivity. The
Pizers write that it is not just giving up a tight hold but, more, recognizing a
breakdown of inner tension between transference and recognition, the tension inherent in the hold of the intrapsychic and the draw of relatedness.
Negotiation is not just consensus building then, the Pizers say, but it is
bridging the intrapsychic and the relational, including transference and the
real, the old and the new, and who in the dyad is doing what to whom. We
bridge outwardly toward the other as we bridge inwardly toward
intrapsychic representations, in Bromberg's terms staying the same while
changing, when we are in the process of negotiating differences with another.

In reviewing the three sessions presented by Levenkron, the Pizers are
able to illustrate this process that is, Holly's negotiation with Ali, in
Holly's actions in bridging the intrapsychic and the relational. The Pizers
demonstrate through examination of the three interactions detailed in
Levenkron's discussion that Holly and Ali are both identified with their
intrapsychic mothers in a complex reverse complementarity. Holly finds
her way out of the entrenched complementarity of maternal identifications, for example, when Holly can hear and register Ali's fear of abandonment as a note of negotiation. The Pizers view Holly's nondisclosure
to Ali of her reasons for canceling sessions as a necessary component in
their two-person dynamic, Holly's personal history assuming a form dic-

tated by the relationship with Ali. As the Pizers put it, Holly "registers the imperative to have a choice about speaking. She doesn't have to agree with Ali's reality of merger and defensive assaults, as she didn't have to agree with her mother's denial of death." In nondisclosing, Holly balanced protecting Ali and protecting herself, an example of Barbara Pizer's concept of intimacy as being oneself with another. The hope, the Pizers say, is that both women—who in their childhoods had had to care for their mothers by not having separate feelings of their own—can join together to feel different in each other's presence.

Conclusion

I end this discussion with much regret that I was unable to do real justice to the richness of these outstanding discussions in consideration of Holly Levenkron's work with Ali. Levenkron has presented us with an exemplary illustration of relational thinking transformed into clinical action, along with an epilogue in which she discusses not only her reactions to the commentaries on her work written by our discussants but also her own reflections on that work written in retrospect.

We learn the specifics of a number of approaches to a relational sensibility from this assemblage, and we are helped to draw a few conclusions about relational work as a whole. First, there is no unified theory of relational thought. Second, there is appreciation for the intersubjective nature of the clinical situation, the intersection of two subjectivities in the field they share, each influencing and responding to the other in ongoing mutuality. Third, attention is given to all modes of communication as they manifest in the dyad. Fourth, there is recognition of the inevitability of self-disclosure—disclosure that is more or less conscious or unconscious and deliberate or inadvertent—and that self-disclosure can be an effective vehicle for change. Fifth, there is the perception that there are multiple forms of intervention in the clinical setting, that interpretation, while still respected, is joined by other forms of being with and responding to the other, including, especially, enactment. Finally, however configured, the importance of the relationship, of two-person, intersubjective interaction, is always regarded as central to clinical work, as opposed to the one-person conceptualization found in the classical model of psychoanalysis.

No doubt there are other generalities inherent in a relational perspective and notable in these discussions, but for the most part even the generalities

I have named are understood and used differently by different analysts with different patients at different times. "Relational" is an attitude, a stance, an understanding—and not a prescription for clinical technique.

I want to conclude by expressing my deep gratitude to all of the contributors in this Issue and for the great opportunity I have been given to edit this assemblage of innovative, indeed pioneering, clinical work.

Estelle Shane, Ph.D.
Issue Editor

Milton Keynes UK
Ingram Content Group UK Ltd.
UKHW040712141024
449569UK00012B/613